MW01256280

This book is considered general health related information and is intended only for healthy adults, ages 18 and older.

The information contained within this book is not meant to diagnose, treat or cure any conditions. You should always seek the guidance of a qualified medical professional before starting any new exercise or diet program.

There may be risks associated with participating in the activities or using products mentioned in this book for people in poor health or with pre-existing medical conditions. If you choose to participate in the activities outlined within you do so willingly and voluntarily and assume all risks associated with these activities.

Specific results mentioned in this book should be considered extraordinary, realizing that there are no "normal" results. Individuals differ drastically as will their results.

Cover Picture by Stephen Herlihy Photography

Cover Design by Logan Herlihy

Edited by Logan Herlihy, Des Marie, & Wende Miner

Published by Amazon Publishing, Inc.

Visit the Author's Website: www.How2LookGoodNaked.com

What People Are Saying About How 2 Look Good Naked:

"I wanted to reach out to you and give you a massive thank you!!! My wife Sara and I started the Keto diet on June 1st after I saw your post on Facebook and requesting a copy of your book "How 2 Look Good Naked". I say diet, but it is more of a lifestyle change. Which sounds bigger and harder, but it really isn't. You do such an incredible job of breaking it down and making it easier to understand. My favorite is how you compare intermediate fasting to running a restaurant, makes perfect sense to me. My wife is down 25lbs and I have dropped about 20lbs. And it's not like other fad diets we have tried where you lose weight quick and it eventually sneaks back. We have both stayed within 2-3lbs without really working out much and cheating a little bit here and there. Dropping the pounds has been great, but more importantly we both feel so much better. More energy, clear headed and a very nice surprise in the bedroom!!! It has definitely brought back a spark in our relationship. We are looking and feeling better naked!!! Thank you!!!"

-Troy & Sara Barfoot, Orlando, FL

"After a debilitating motorcycle accident, I gained quite a bit of weight and struggled to lose it or keep it off. There are so many fad diets, so many supplements, little tips and tricks that everyone and their mother seems to being trying to pawn off on you. None of them work because all of them market their 'program' as just that: a program. Something you can do to get to where you want and then go back to your unhealthy habits. There are no quick fixes. Anything that you plan on quitting once you've hit some imaginary goal isn't going to work long term. What Logan puts forth here is such a breath of fresh air. Rather than implementing some unrealistic or unhealthy master plan, this book is just about creating a life that you can enjoy and look good doing it. If you want to look good and feel good, all while getting to continue doing the things you enjoy, then read this book."

-Tyler J. Rits

"Was fat now not fat. Book good."

-Albert Einstein

<u>Acknowledgements:</u>

The biggest takeaway from this whole experience might be to always be kind to and keep in contact with your old college drinking buddies. This whole process has just been a never ending marathon of going back and tinkering. Nothing I've ever written before whether for business or pleasure has ever been so painstakingly torn apart. I've had hugely successful blogs, countless A+ papers and essays for school, almost none of them did I give more than a simple once over. I have always been a firm believer that whatever grammatical errors may express themselves, are not nearly as important as the content and the core of the message I'm trying to convey.

While I still firmly and wholeheartedly believe that, that's unfortunately just not acceptable when it comes to publishing. Honest mistakes will happen, but not without first going over everything in depth with a fine tooth comb (which I find about as enjoyable as having fingernails plucked out with rusty tweezers). So thank goodness for friends and loved ones willing to do all the fine tooth combing that I tried to but after a certain point could simply not bring myself to do anymore.

Thank you to Des Marie for my initial round of edits and encouraging me that this was something worth reading. To Wende Miner for really digging in and challenging me to simplify and make sense of some of the more complex topics covered. And finally, to Tyler Rits, my college drinking bro who surfaced out of nowhere with insights and a helping hand I will be forever indebted to. It took a lot of work (that I didn't want to do) to get this book in your hands. The writing is the easy part, it's making sense of it all that takes some time.

"The best time to plant a tree was 20 years ago; the second best time is NOW."

-Chinese Proverb

How 2 Look Good Naked

The Least Amount of Effort, To Look The Best With Your Clothes Off

----

Logan Emmett Herlihy

CONTENTS:

INTRODUCTION

Let's just go ahead and get this out there. This is not going to be your typical health and wellness book. I'm not going to tell you why everything else is garbage and this and _only this_ is the way to a better, more ideal you, because quite frankly, it's not. There are plenty of diets and plenty of routines that work for _plenty_ of people. What this is, is my experience, plain and simple - The best, easiest and most effective ways I've found to lose weight, feel good, and, most importantly, look good.

We will not be trying to achieve a "Spartan Physique". There is no "Superhero Method" and honestly, I couldn't tell you what the F*&K the movie stars do, because I don't have endless amounts of free time, money, and people telling me what to do and how to do it. I will not be only offering my beginner tips to get you in the door, and then offering ongoing "Platinum" service for just $29.99/month.

This will simply be my experience over the past few years. Specifically, what I have found to be the safest, easiest, and most effective ways to get the body in which I feel comfortable. Some people want to get big, hard, ripped, (insert Men's Health adjective) muscles. Many people want promises of shredded abs, and sculpted thighs. Honestly, I'm tired of all that and I'm fresh out of buzzwords. Contained in this book you'll find a simple way to live, feel, and look better. I'll give you the basics of what's worked for me and helped me achieve the results I've always wanted. All it takes is a little bit of effort, a willingness to improve, and a dash of self-control.

If that doesn't seem too unreasonable, then take a few days, browse through this book, and pick out what you think will work for you.

Try something. If that works, then try the next thing, and so on and so forth. In my experience trying to change too much, too quickly, only leads to frustration, excuses, and eventually giving up. Don't give up, go slow! Some of this stuff takes some getting used to, but when your body adapts, you will see changes, slowly at first, and pretty drastically the longer you keep with it. You may be asking how did this whole H.2.L.G.N. thing come about, well, I'll tell you.

My Story

I spent years and years as a five to six times a week gym rat. I'd be lying if I said I didn't have better than average genetics, but I did a lot of work to try to make myself even better. I've tried eating clean, eating six small meals a day, going vegetarian, and pescatarian, and even vegan-light. But I could never shake those last few pounds.

Even when I was in my best shape, following my best diet, I always felt like I could achieve more. Part of what I hope to help you accomplish with this book is realizing that measuring yourself by someone else's standards will always leave you longing for more. It wasn't until I started experimenting with this program, paying attention to not just what, but *when* I ate, and getting the gym rat mentality out of my head, that I made massive amounts of progress.

This isn't a fitness and nutrition program I spent massive amounts of time developing, it honestly just kind of fell into my lap. I got the right job, at the right time, at the right place in my life. I no longer had hours to spend at the gym every day (even though I was working at a gym), and the first thing that became apparent to me was I would need to start keeping better watch of my diet. The gym I worked at were proponents of Ketogenic Diets. I read a lot about Ketogenics, I tried some things, and they worked. I tried some other things, and they didn't work.

I was seeing that weight was dropping off, but I assumed that this had something to do with the fact that I could only make time to work out (maybe) twice a week. With the benefit of the gym I was at, and the modality we prescribed to, I made the most of my limited workout time. My one to two 20-minute sessions per week were absolutely grueling and physically more taxing than almost anything I had done before. Slowly, more things started to happen.

I began to hone in on my dietary choices. I started cooking more for myself and doing more research into recipes. I was okay with sacrificing certain things, but I refused to eat nothing but chicken breasts and asparagus. I found that weight kept coming off, to the point where I almost began to worry that maybe I was going too far. With tracking at my gym however, I noticed that my strength was not just staying the same... it was increasing, and drastically.

Every few weeks I would hear something new about diet or exercise, and try it out. I listened to a lot of podcasts, I read a lot of blogs, and I kept tweaking and fine tuning. The result is what you will see in the following pages. What you can expect is probably something similar to what I experienced. Using this book as your jumping off point, taking some concepts, trying out a few ideas, and then seeing results. Then doing even more research and creating your own program based on your own body and experience.

There's a few things in here that I think should be followed no matter what, and they will be laid out that way. The rest is basically a "choose your own adventure" story. I can't promise everything will go exactly for you the way it did for me, but this is what I have experienced over the last 12 months. In the beginning of 2017 I weighed close to 200 pounds (195-198 most days) with a body fat percentage around 20%. I now regularly weigh between 160-165 pounds, and my body fat is now below 8% consistently.

The important thing to remember here, is losing weight was never what I set out to do. A few pounds maybe, but not upwards of 30 lbs and 10% body fat. The other thing I don't want to be forgotten here is, I do not starve myself, I eat... a lot. But what I eat, and again more importantly, *when* I eat has continued to change drastically. A final important thing to remember here is the fact that I've lost *no strength* during all this. And when I say I've gotten stronger I don't mean simply in relation to my strength/weight ratio (which has skyrocketed), I mean I'm actually stronger than I've ever been.

So what can you expect? Expect to feel a little weird. Expect to feel a little hungry (at first). Expect to learn a little bit about a lot of different topics covering nutrition and fitness. If you've never worked out before, expect to be sore. If you are or used to be a gym rat, expect to question how in the world you can expect to see results working out twice a week. Expect to want to continue to do some research of your own, beyond what I've done. Expect to start feeling better, then start hearing that you're looking better. Expect that to motivate you to do a little bit more each day.

Expect that sometimes the scale lies to you, but the mirror always tells the brutally honest truth. Expect to get to a point where the methods outlined in this book become second nature, where you don't have to actively think about how long it's been since you've eaten, or if you've worked out this week. Expect it to become intuitive. Expect to say to yourself (quite often), "I think I made too much food." And then expect to eat it all anyways. Expect to look good, real good, totally naked.

How 2 Look Good Naked, is just that, a guide to being comfortable in your own skin. I don't claim to know everything, but I am a nationally certified personal trainer, and I've got close to 3,000 one-on-one training sessions under my belt. So I do have some idea. If you're willing to take the journey then I'm excited to help start you on the right path.

Your Pal in Fitness,
Logan Herlihy

PART I:

GETTING STARTED

<u>What Does It Mean To Be Healthy?</u>

Before we try to embark on this journey of change and self-exploration, we have to establish some ground rules. As I stated in the introduction, this is not a fad diet or workout program. I spent too many years of my life trying to fit and mold my body one way or another, and at the end of a decade of running myself into the ground, I finally settled on two elements of fitness I won't compromise on:

#1: I want to feel great

#2: I want to look good

Now the order and wording of those two are important, and something I struggled with for many years. Some of you my be thinking, "The book is called 'How 2 Look Good Naked', so why is 'Feel Great' listed first"? After a long, challenging road to get here what I've learned is that the easiest way to start the journey to looking good is to feel good *first*. Change how you feel on a day to day basis and focus on that. Eventually how you look will start to reflect how you feel.

This is why #1 is vastly more important than #2, and that it has everything to do with what it means to be healthy. For many people, especially those peddling lifestyle advice in the fitness industry, #2 is at the top of the list, and those adjectives "good" and "great" are also flip-flopped. We are led to believe that we can achieve all the happiness in the world, contingent upon one little thing... that you must always look AMAZING, 100% of the time.

However, most people don't actually care about getting or maintaining a six-pack. They simply want to feel better on a daily basis. My hope with following the program outlined in these pages is that regardless of what your goals are physically, you will start to feel better, and eventually you will reach and eclipse any physical goals you thought possible.

The other part of the problem with mixing up those two elements is that you can look great, and feel like shit... all the time. There are many forms of this, but from my own personal experience, I would always sacrifice how I felt always in favor of what I wanted to look like. It didn't matter if I was hungover, sick, heartbroken, I was going to the gym, five times a week, no matter what. I also was able to explain and justify poor diet and life decisions because I knew that I could just "work it off". I slept like shit, I ate like shit, and most importantly, most of the time, I felt like shit... but I looked great... I thought.

The eureka moment I had in my fitness journey was when I decided I would flip my priorities. I would make *feeling great* the main focus, and looking good would hopefully be a realistic outcome because of it... and it worked. This is why #1 on my list (feeling great) is and always will be vastly more important than #2 (looking good), because I can do #2 without doing #1, but I can't do #1 without doing #2. This book could really be called: "How 2 Feel Great Naked, Which In Time Will Lead To You Looking Better, And Eventually Help You Look Good Naked Too". But that's not quite as catchy...

So what does it mean to be healthy?

There are lots of different ways we could define this, diving into physiology and nutrition (and we will to some extent), but I want you to think about it this way. Healthy for the purposes of this book simply means feeling great. Healthy means going to sleep at night without having to quiet your mind. It means waking up in the morning and not feeling groggy or sleep deprived. Healthy is enjoying a cup of coffee, but not needing it to function.

Thinking clearly, and being able to make it through your work day without aches and pains. Healthy is enjoying good food, not portion controlling, and not pigging out. Healthy is rewarding yourself when you've earned it, and not feeling guilty about slipping up. It means looking forward to physical challenges and activities, and not viewing exercise as a burden. So ask yourself this question... are you healthy?

As we start to embark on the different ideas and activities outlined in this book, I want you to always keep that idea of feeling great in the back of your mind. There is no one size fits all fitness or diet solution for everyone, we are all WAY too different. Some people can eat vegan and feel great, others get physically sick from eating only fruits and vegetables. It's not because they don't want it enough, they are simply built differently. That's why the way you feel is the most important thing of which you should be aware.

The truth is when you start incorporating these ideas I'm going to lay out, you might not *feel* great at first, but bear with me for a little and see if the way you feel doesn't start to change. If you've never paid attention to the food you've put in your body before and the way you've exercised, then it makes sense that you wouldn't be in tune with the natural messages your body sends you. We're so over-saturated with garbage all the time, that feeling sluggish and dragging is, for many of us, our natural state. But when we start to make incremental changes, we begin to feel our energy levels changing, our mood starts to stabilize, and to some extent our old habits and cravings start to slip away.

If I had tried to implement all of the things I do on a daily basis now all at once five years ago, I wouldn't have lasted a week. It seems extreme. That's why the plan I will outline for you in this book goes in phases. We'll start easy. I don't expect you to just start out fasting for 16-20 hours at a time, especially if you haven't changed your diet at all. You'll go insane. But you can start with 12 hours (no eating two hours before bed, sleep 8, skip breakfast... boom 12 hours). The best part about going slowly, especially with the processes I've learned over the years, is that you'll still see results. Simply by being cognizant of *when and what* you're eating is enough for many to start noticing a difference in how they approach their health.

Just remember what I said in the introduction: baby steps. Try something, and if it works, take the next step. If you find you can't handle the next step, but you were having success with the previous step, take a step back and stick with what works for you. Like I said, everyone is built differently. Some will be able to easily incorporate all these ideas and see great results, others may struggle with the deeper program, but everyone can benefit from a couple of small changes in lifestyle. The real key is focusing on how you start to feel as you continue. If you start feeling better, you'll start looking better, and pretty soon you'll be more comfortable being naked than a toddler in a tub!

Where Do I Start?

Let's be clear here... this is not a total-body crazy cleanse and life changing pyramid-scheme. There is not magic juicing shake, and no one-on-one life coaching sessions. This is all about you, and what *you* want to accomplish. That being said, the subtitle of this book is "The *Least* Amount of Effort to Look the Best With Your Clothes Off." The emphasis here is on *least* amount of effort. To get going on this program you don't need a gym membership, or a recipe guide, or really any outside utilities. You can simply start. As you progress, you'll notice we'll start to add in some recommendations (finding a gym, starting to cook for yourself, etc.) but for now you don't need anything except this book to get started. If you're ready, let's begin... seriously... right now.

Assignment #1:

Starting now, and going until you finish reading this book (which shouldn't take very long, but let's assume you stretch it out to a week) I want you to just **be acutely aware of your eating timetable each day**. What does that mean to you? If you want to write it down, that's great. If not, don't bother, but just make an active effort to think about when you're eating each day. Not how much, mind you, just when. Do you eat over the course of eight hours? Ten hours? 18 hours? Are you eating non-stop (snacking) from the second you wake up to the second you pass out? Don't worry about what that means for you yet, just become aware. It doesn't get much easier than that, so congrats... you've started! Did you just lose a pound?

For most people the idea of paying attention to when you eat isn't typically part of a normal day, so simply by becoming aware of when you are eating you will have a leg up. Think of it as a food-inspired meditation practicing "presence". Think about it when you have breakfast in the morning, whenever you grab a snack (even that bite size snickers... that counts), dinner, late night munchies, just be aware.

If you do just that, you would undoubtedly see results in the course of your lifetime, because the truth is, most of us are not aware when we are eating. If we were, we would be much more careful about what it was, when it was, and how much it was. My focus is simplicity, but I want to give you a broader picture of what that means. I'm sure some of you have been thinking that when I say the "least" amount of effort I mean that as a subjective term.

"Ya, that's probably easy for him, but it's gotta be crazy for anyone else!"

But actually, I mean "least" in the most objective way possible, especially compared to other things I've tried in the past. In case you have any misconceptions that I may be trying to sneak some crazy ideas in here, I'll tell you what the "least" amount of effort looks like for me in my daily life.

THINGS I DON'T DO IN MY DIET:

- *I don't count calories*
- *I don't count carbohydrates*
- *I don't actively count macronutrients*
- *I don't worry about cheating (more on this later)*
- *I don't stay away from restaurants*
- *I don't starve myself*
- *I don't weigh my portions (or myself)*
- *I don't feel bad*

THINGS I DON'T DO IN MY EXERCISE ROUTINE:

- *I don't work out more than twice a week*
- *I don't spend more than 40 minutes exercising at one time*
- *I don't feel bad if I miss a day*
- *I don't dread going to the gym*
- *I don't worry about my weight*
- *I don't do "cardio" (a lot more about this later)*
- *I don't take 1,000 different supplements (i.e. Pre-Workout, BCAA's, 1,000 grams of Protein/day, etc.)*
- *I don't... and I can't stress this enough... I DON'T CARE what other people are doing in the gym*

You may be asking yourself, "if I don't do any of those things... what do I do?". The answer is pretty obvious isn't it... the *least* amount possible, to feel the best I've ever felt. Now that you have started Assignment 1, and you know what I do and don't do, let's start looking at what you can expect.

What Can You Expect?

This is going to be a little bit different than anything else you've tried before. This isn't a 30-day all or nothing challenge. What I'm going to try to do is slowly change the way you look at diet and exercise to allow you the easiest way to make progress, and maintain it. In this process you will get out what you put in. If you incorporate all these suggestions right away, you'll notice immediate changes. If you decide to go the slow and steady route, expect seeing results will take a bit longer.

What I'd like to see is for you to find something that works for you, using this as simply the outline and then making your own decisions for your life. If you do everything I do, the way I do it, you can expect to see some drastic changes. But even by just being more aware of what you do on a day-to-day basis, you'll notice progress. I've sent this book to about 50 or so people over the course of getting it ready for publication, and here's one on my favorite reactions so far. For more results and stories like this be sure to visit my website

www.How2LookGoodNaked.com

Logan,

I wanted to reach out to you and give you a massive thank you!!! My wife Sara and I started the Keto diet on June 1st after I saw your post on Facebook and requesting a copy of your book "How to look good naked". I say diet, but it is more of a lifestyle change. Which sounds bigger and harder, but it really isn't. You do such an incredible job of breaking it down and making it easier to understand. My favorite is how you compare intermediate fasting to running a restaurant, makes perfect sense to me.

My wife is down 25lbs and I have dropped about 20lbs. And it's not like other fad diets we have tried where you lose weight quick and it eventually sneaks back. We have both stayed within 2-3lbs without really working out much and cheating a little bit here and there. Dropping the pounds has been great, but more importantly we both feel so much better. More energy, clear headed and a very nice surprise in the bedroom!!! It has definitely brought back a spark in our relationship. We are looking and feeling better naked!!! Thank you!!!

One more result I would like to share, I have always had very high triglycerides (663 last tested, normal high is 150). That test also put me in a "pre-diabetic" category and high risk for heart disease. That woke me up, I did not want to go on their drugs that I would have to take for the rest of my life. Drugs that wouldn't fix the problem and would also cause even more issues. I recently was tested again after being Keto for 4 months and my results were amazing, 298. Still higher than desired, but a huge improvement.

I know this diet goes against everything we have been taught our entire lives... but it works! It is not hard and once you start feeling the difference in how great your body feels you stop missing and craving carbs. It is a lot of fun trying new Keto recipes and as you mention in the book, its ok to cheat a little here and there without gaining weight back. It is surprisingly easy to keep it off. And when you cheat, you will notice a difference in how your body feels... and it makes you not really want to cheat.

Thank you so much Logan! Your book was very inspiring and full of knowledge that was a pleasure to read with action steps that are easy to follow through with. Keep on spreading the good word and making the world feel great naked!

Sincerely,

Troy and Sara Barfoot

PART II:

BACK TO BASICS

What's Most Important? (Surprise, it's Diet)

As much as this may surprise you, there is no such thing as six-pack abs from an "Ab-stimulator"- don't believe the Facebook ads. I feel completely confident in saying that no one has ever gone from a beer belly to a rock-hard six-pack by sticking electrodes to their gut and waiting for the miracle to happen. The miracle, unfortunately, does not exist. It's pretty straight forward and always has been. I've heard the cliché and hated it, but the honest truth is this: "Fitness starts in the Kitchen". This book does not have the time or scope to go into the *vast* enterprise of proper diet and nutrition. What I can do, however, is cover some of the basics of what we do know about diet, and dispel some common misconceptions that are pervasive in our culture.

There is new and exciting science behind the type of dieting we will be adhering to which will make your weight loss and fitness goals finally within reach. The reality is, there is no *one diet* that works for everyone. It doesn't exist, and anyone who claims to have a one-size-fits-all diet is probably lying to you. We all have evolved over generations to have similar fundamental dietary needs: essential fats, minerals, etc. However, the types of these needs and the way we can go about optimally fulfilling them is very different.

Diet and Nutrition is a constantly evolving field, where new mechanisms and cause and effect relationships are being discovered all the time. What we know and understand today is vastly different than even five or ten years ago, and that information is drastically different than what we thought we understood two and three decades ago. For years, dairy and grains were foundational parts of the food pyramid and the backbone of foundational principles of diet and nutrition. Specifically in the last decade, the field of nutrition has made great strides in understanding how our bodies react with certain food groups, and now gluten and dairy are among its top offenders for allergies, disease correlation, and overall unhealthy foods for the masses.

The point is this: listening to our bodies is the most valuable tool we have when it comes to overall dietary health. If working with an Registered Dietician or Nutritionist is something you're interested in, just be sure you find someone whose practice is evolving with the current scientific knowledge.

So Why is Diet So Important?

We need to change the way we think about our relationship with food. The first step to that is the first assignment I've tasked you with in this book, becoming aware of *when* we are eating. We'll also add **Assignment #2: becoming aware of *what* you're eating.** These two things will have huge impacts as we experiment with the diet plan laid out in the upcoming chapters and will help you as you grow and adapt your diet to your own personal needs.

This is diet as referring to lifestyle, not just changing what or how we eat for the purpose of a short and drastic change in our bodies, but changing our relationship with what and how we eat for the rest of our lives. This will not be a temporary diet that you go on, but will be a fundamental change to your diet in terms of the food you habitually eat.

The reason diet is so important to overall health and wellness is because for the past few hundred generations of mankind, what and when they ate was how they survived. Before the agricultural revolution and the advent of mass food production, human beings were dependent on their environment and their diet for survival. Though it seems like there has never been a time without energy drinks, protein shakes, and Kombucha, for most of human history we survived and thrived without the help of outside supplementation. Over the course of evolution, this has made the human body one of the most well suited and adaptive organisms on the planet, but with advancement has come sedation.

Our bodies are set up to thrive in the right conditions, and if we can produce those conditions, they can run more efficiently. Food is fuel, plain and simple. If properly chosen and managed it can give our bodies all the tools it needs to operate at maximum efficiency, no supplements needed. Now this is not to say that supplementation cannot offer a boost, because it can. But putting premium gas in a lemon doesn't change the fact that it's a lemon. If we treat our bodies with proper diet and nutrition like the high-performance machines they are, then we can expect to see even more results with extra supplementation. But all the supplements in the world will not improve a body with no efficiency.

With the new understanding of diet fundamentals outlined in this book, and working to find out exactly what type of diet works best for you, you will be amazed at how efficient your own body is. The problem many of us have is we are so bogged down with years of poor maintenance that it's all our bodies can do to simply hold the line. We are not meant to struggle to stay at equilibrium, we as human beings are meant to thrive. However, unless you've experienced what this feels like first hand, you probably don't know the capabilities your own body actually holds. As we start to clear away some of the wreckage of the past, you will begin to notice how your body is no longer just "maintaining", but optimizing.

Until we clear out the years, and sometimes decades worth of buildup however, supplements don't offer us much of an advantage. The typical American Diet leaves you with huge deficiencies that cannot be overcome by supplementing alone. Let's clear out some of this gunk in the engine... then we can talk about adding a NOS tank.

Reintroduction to Dieting

Remember when we are referring to diet here, we're talking about the things we *habitually eat*. This is not a short-sighted change in what we're taking into our bodies simply to jump start metabolism and then go back to eating poorly later. There are no "secret" fat burning foods, and anyone claiming to know of such a food is full of it. This is a reorganization and new understanding of what eating is supposed to look like. Many times in fad diets the emphasis is on *what* we eat. Many diets falsely advertise that simply by changing the *what* (i.e. greens and organics) we can see a complete turnaround.

These claims are false. The *what* is obviously extremely important, because we're not going to be running at maximum efficiency if all we're eating is Twinkies and Taco Bell. However, per "Assignment #1" I want to introduce something that is foreign to most people when it comes to changing dietary habits. In my experience this approach has been vastly more influential on overall health and weight loss, and that's examining *when* we eat.

What is Intermittent Fasting (IMF)?

At its most basic level, IMF is keeping a running total of the time throughout the day in which we are actively eating and taking in calories, and when we are not. Although the finer points of IMF are up for debate, almost everyone who is a proponent of this dietary style agrees you must fast for at least 12 hours to be considered practicing IMF. In my experience with IMF I've gone from 12 hours to upwards of 22 hours between meals. In the following sections I'll discuss what types of fasting I've found to be most beneficial.

Research has shown that changing eating timetables alone and incorporating fasting periods of 12 plus hours can have massive benefits on multiple levels. Improved weight loss efficiency, mood, sleep behavioral patterns, and disease prevention are just a few of the many proclaimed benefits of IMF. The real key however, is fasting increases insulin sensitivity, and opens up the bodies availability to focus on things besides digestion, which is not the case when we eat every 3-4 hours.

But rather than delve too deeply into why and how all these benefits arise, we are simply going to build upon the idea that: *Fasting for at least 12 hours a day has benefits for overall health and wellness.* An idea that is pretty widely accepted in the scientific community. The validity of disease prevention, mood stabilization and others, are linked, but not beyond the realm of criticism and differing opinions. So instead of making bold extravagant claims for the purpose of this book we will operate under this broad idea: "Fasting for at least 12 hours per day has benefits to overall health and wellness."

Going forward we are going to use this idea of a 12-hour eating time frame or "window" and build from there. This is the first example of one of our cornerstones, the absolute least you can do for your diet and still see results (slowly, but surely). That being said this one is non-negotiable. There is no reason any of us can't be expected (at the very least) to keep our daily eating schedule within a 12-hour time frame. And as you will see as the layers continue to build, this idea of 12-hours becomes more important and fundamental to doing as little as possible to feel great and look good.

We'll also be exploring the *what* we're eating per **Assignment #2.** The *when* is arguably more important, but there is no doubt that eating healthy, satiating foods is supremely important for sustained success with any diet. We'll dive a lot deeper into these topics, but I first want to outline some of the ideas we'll be covering. This is not the only way to eat, but these are the methods I have found easiest to incorporate and use to sustain long-term commitment and happiness with my own diet. While we could argue the finer points of meat or no meat, for the purposes of this book we will be practicing a omnivorous diet (meat and plants). There are many ways you can modify for meat substitutes, whether for health or ethical reasons. What I ask is that rather than disparaging based on beliefs, you simply key in on the overall ideas laid out here, and work out your own guidelines as you begin your journey.

Dietary Ideas and Outlines for H.2.L.G.N.

- *Introduction to Ketosis, and basic Ketogenic Ideas.*
- *Dispelling some commonly accepted misinformation among dieting practices.*
- *Lowering our daily carbohydrate intake, instead using fat for fuel.*
- *Starting with a 12-hour eating window, eventually working down to an ideal 4-8 hour window.*
- *Introducing how adding grass fed butter and MCT oil to our morning coffee can assist (without affecting) the fasting process*
- *Exploring the gut biome and the intestinal circadian rhythm (and how that fits in with fasting).*
- *Working towards a 9-12 hour window within the constraints of the intestinal circadian rhythm.*

If none of that makes any sense to you... fear not! We will continue to explore these ideas more deeply in the next two sections of Part II. Our goal is to have a very broad understanding of the mechanisms of the inner workings of our body, and my hope is a deeper appreciation for controlling our eating habits. You will not be a certified dietary expert after finishing this section, but you will have all the tools needed to continue to do your own research and delve further into these ideas as you would like.

The Subtle Art of Not Starving Yourself

It's time to really delve into the "what" we're eating, and to change what our diet looks like, by changing the types of foods we habitually eat. This isn't a "restrictive" diet, but we will be trying to restrict certain types of foods. Foods that we either know have little to no nutritional benefit, or foods that simply are counterproductive to the metabolic changes we will attempt to make in our bodies. This is where the *what we eat* of **Assignment #2** really starts to come into play.

I told you in the beginning of this book that I *don't count calories*, and that's true, but that doesn't mean I just eat whatever I want. I do eat whatever I want, as long as that *whatever* fulfills certain dietary guidelines. To understand this a little bit better we have to go a little deeper into our understanding of "food as fuel". As with everything else in this book, I will spare you the physiological in-depth analysis and try to pair this down to just the basics.

Exploring "Ketosis" (Fat for Fuel)

Ketosis is something that occurs naturally in our bodies when we have limited the amount of glucose available to burn as energy. In a ketogenic state the body reverts to burning fat as "fuel" for the normal daily metabolic processes. In layman's terms what this means is when we limit carbohydrates in our daily diet (usually less than 20-100 net carbs) our body is forced to burn our fat stores in their place. But getting into and maintaining ketosis is much more than simply getting on a "low-carb" diet.

In doing research for this book I studied the old food pyramid, and the new "My Plate" (released in 2011). In both cases (the pyramid and the plate) the recommended daily make up of simple and complex carbohydrates is in the 40-65% ballpark. Though these standards and guidelines are not embraced by many in the dietary and nutritional community, it doesn't change the fact that this is what the vast majority of Americans are exposed to. Though traditional humans had the capabilities to process carbs when they were available, most research suggests our ancestors were taking in significantly less carbohydrates on average, and those carbs were most certainly unprocessed.

Okay, so why is this little social history lesson important, and what does it have to do with the new diet we are trying to undertake in H.2.L.G.N.? The reason understanding the history of carbohydrates in the modern diet is important, is because many of us (myself included) were wrongly led to believe that carbs are the only type of sustainable energy we can use. When I was studying physiology in school there was always talk of simple vs. complex carbs, the way they are processed in our bodies, and the difference in levels of sustained energy. What they failed to mention, and what I didn't know until beginning my own fitness journey, is that there is another, *far* more effective form of food as fuel for human beings... fat.

Why Fat Instead of Carbohydrates?

Standards expressed in the food pyramid (2005), say the average person should consume somewhere in the ballpark of 2,000 calories/day. Of those calories 40-65% should come from carbohydrates. This equates to a baffling 200-325 grams of carbohydrates per day! But this type of dietary setup assumes that many of us live an active enough lifestyle that we can realistically burn hundreds of carbohydrates per day. For most of us this is not the case.

As we try to incorporate doing as little as possible to feel and look as good as possible, consuming 100's of carbs daily is not ideal. In fact, it's counterproductive. Left to sit idle, carbohydrates raise insulin levels and eventually become part of the fat stores which we are already trying to actively chip away. This is where Ketosis becomes important.

When limiting carbohydrates and converting to a low-carb, high-fat diet, we are essentially replacing what we are burning. After a certain amount of time rewiring our bodies, we can become fat burning machines. Along with this idea of using fat as fuel we will also additionally add on multiple layers of other body hacks to maximize our body's efficiency. When we eventually get to a state where we are regularly burning fat instead of carbohydrates, you will begin to see where the ideas of "limiting" the amount of food we eat for a diet starts to fall apart.

The best analogy I've found for this is Kindling vs. Charcoal. Our bodies react to carbs much like a fire reacts to kindling. It's an immediate energy source that provides a big spark, but also burns out extremely fast. Fat on the other hand reacts much more like Charcoal. It's a little harder to get going, but once it does it provide a long steady burn that last for hours.

Getting Started with Keto

One of the important things to remember as we continue to progress through this new program is that there are stages. If you want to attempt to immediately cut out carbohydrates totally from your diet and replace all your foods with high-fat and moderate-protein options... good luck. For many, this is the hardest part. If you've never taken the time to look at the nutrition labels on some of the food you consume on a regular basis, then do so. You might be shocked to see just how pervasive carbohydrates are in basically everything consumed with regularity in America. From energy drinks packed with sugar, down to "healthy snacks" regularly marketed as low-fat alternatives. Carbs are *everywhere!*

As you continue with your first two assignments in this journey (being aware of what and when we eat), let's add on **Assignment #3: start looking at carbohydrates in the food you regularly consume.** Attempt to keep a running mental total throughout the day, or if you feel so inclined, write it down. I think most people would be shocked at how regularly we consume massive amounts of carbohydrates at each sitting. This becomes especially true when we eat out at restaurants. Though many restaurants have adopted calorie counts available on menus, many don't provide a nutritional breakdown of items unless you ask specifically to see it. So now you have 3 assignments:

- **Assignment #1: Pay attention to *when* you eat.**
- **Assignment #2: Pay attention to *what* you eat.**
- **Assignment #3: Pay attention to the *carbohydrates* you eat.**

This is now your checklist of things to do before we even attempt to start changing our habitual eating habits.

What's important is not biting off more than we can chew (pun intended). For many of us carbohydrates, converted in our bodies to glucose, have been the *only* form of bodily energy we've ever known. When we begin to start limiting our carbohydrate intake many will experience something known as the "Keto Flu". Essentially your body's adjustment period to reorganizing the way we gain and synthesize energy, and you may feel like *shit!*

This will be especially true as we begin to whittle away at one of the most notorious offenders of carbohydrates in the modern diet... sugar. Headaches, nausea, sweats, these are the things that are typical as we turn our bodies from garbage processing plants into high functioning machinery, and they suck... but, this too shall pass.

The next part of this section we will be exploring another compounding layer that goes in compliment with this new Ketogenic Diet. It's something we've discussed a little already, Intermittent Fasting. We'll explore how we can "hack" this idea and use it to our advantage, without feeling like we're starving ourselves. We'll also look into how combining this with a high-fat diet can compound our results, and help us stay on track and motivated.

Combining Intermittent Fasting and Ketosis

We've now covered the *what* and the *when* we discussed earlier in this book, and you've been working on Assignments 1, 2, and 3. Now let's take your observations and the previous ideas and tie them together, creating a picture of what your H.2.L.G.N. daily life will look like.

So, we now know that Intermittent Fasting has massive benefits. We also know that by switching to a Ketogenic Diet we can start using fat for fuel. But how can we use these ideas in unison to compound the results of both? One of the most transformative pieces of information I have found was from Dave Asprey.

Asprey is a self-proclaimed "biohacker" and Founder of BulletProof©, a supplement and nutritional company who's been instrumental in challenging many mainstream ideas about nutrition. While Asprey makes many grandiose claims (without sufficient research), I believe he does so in the hopes of promoting self-awareness. Helping people to realize there are many more efficient ways to run the machine that is our bodies, you just have to find them.

One of Asprey's initial findings which led him along his journey to becoming the king of "bio-hackers" was something he calls BulletProof Coffee©. Essentially, this is taking high quality, mold free coffee, and adding grass-fed butter, and MCT Oil (medium chain triglycerides). What that means is combining coffee with "healthy fats". The reasoning for this is two-fold.

#1: *Quality coffee allows you to kick start your brain*: Much of the coffee on the market of lesser quality is exposed to mold toxins. This creates the brain crash you typically feel after drinking coffee. Especially while fasting we need our brains at 100%.

#2: *Adding healthy fats allows us to "cheat" Intermittent Fasting*: The principle here being that once we've started to make the shift to a fat-burning state, adding *just fat* into our bodies (the way coffee with butter and MCT does) won't dilute the value we gain from fasting. Instead because it is pure fat our body takes it in stride, and this allows us to fast for vastly longer periods comfortably. This is because the fat keeps us satiated, even though we have not yet *officially* eaten anything.

Drinking coffee with grass fed butter and MCT oil while Intermittent Fasting, makes it much easier to handle the extended fasting periods (In a later section we'll look at my own twist on Dave's recipe, I call *Naked Coffee).* This however, does not grant us free reign to fill our coffee full of as much fat as we would like (remember, it is calorie dense). What we want to gain with this combination is simply the ability to extend our fasting time without mentally or physically crashing.

Before we can totally tie Ketosis and IMF together, I want to introduce two more concepts that will be of utmost importance. Without going too deeply into the physiology, it's important to understand a little bit more about our guts, and how we can assist them to make our bodies fat burning machines.

I would encourage everyone who reads this book to do more research on the gut biome and something coined the "Mind-Gut Connection". I was first exposed to this idea by Dr. Kelly Brogan. Brogan is an amazing scientist, author, and homeopathic health advocate. She explains this connection far more eloquently than I, but I will try. The gut of the human body is an extremely important and complex part of our anatomy which is often overlooked in modern health and wellness. As the field of nutrition has continued to advance and update its ideas in the last few decades, the importance of the gut has taken a center stage in mainstream health and wellness. Basically, what the "Mind-Gut Connection" is all about is that taking care of our gut health will have a slew of other benefits on our mental and physical state. Essentially, "eat better, feel better".

Among a wide range of things we have now come to know about the gut, one in particular stands out. An idea that helps in understanding and explaining this connection between diet and fasting. It's something another brilliant researcher Dr. Rhonda Patrick refers to as our gut's "circadian rhythm". A circadian rhythm, as it is most commonly referenced in day-to-day life, refers to our body's natural sleep patterns. We have a natural process we go through on a daily basis from before we wake up, right up until we close our eyes to sleep at night. This rhythm is basically a cycle which helps us rise to our day, be at our most alert through the important parts, and then wind back down again at night to achieve sleep, rejuvenate and do it all over again. Dr. Patrick postulates from a plethora of scientific studies that our gut works in much the same way, with a natural cycle of time for function, and time for recuperation.

Essentially, when our gut is "turned on" in the morning, most commonly from the first thing we eat or drink that is not water, our gut's "internal clock" starts to tick. Even with the introduction of our morning cup of coffee, our bodies begin producing time sensitive enzymes. These enzymes begin the process of breaking down and processing all the nutrients and minerals we take into our body that day. These enzymes are essentially on a timer that runs out after 12-hours. Our gut has done its work for the day, and now it wants to take some much-deserved time off. But what happens if we just keep eating?

Similar to our normal sleep schedule, if you just continue to stay awake and don't allow yourself to sleep, things start to go wrong... and fast. The best way I know how to simplify the in-depth way that Dr. Patrick introduced these ideas is through an analogy as follows. Imagine that your gut is like a restaurant. This restaurant is open from noon-midnight each day (12-hours) and operates on a very tight and time efficient schedule.

Let's assume throughout the course of an ideal day things run as such. At noon the doors open and a relatively few number of customers come in. These customers are light eaters and low maintenance. They put very little pressure on the staff of the restaurant, which allows them time to prepare for their typical lunch and dinner rushes.

At 2pm the lunch rush arrives. Having more than enough time to prepare, the kitchen and waitstaff run easily and efficiently. Everyone's job is done just as it should and when it should. The rush comes and goes and now the entire staff once again has time to prepare for the evening's normal dinner rush.

At 7pm the dinner rush arrives. Much like the lunch rush, having had plenty of time to prepare, the staff works as if a well-oiled machine. All the customers are taken care of efficiently and easily, and as usual the customers begin to wind down around 9pm. Being that this is an *ideal* day, the waitstaff knows that they can now begin to prepare the restaurant for the next day.

They begin to clean their sections both on the floor and in the kitchen, leaving just enough waitstaff out to deal with any unforeseen late night guests, even though no such guests show. The restaurant is fully cleaned and ready for another successful day. The staff closes the doors at midnight and is entirely out the door by 12:01, another perfect day. This is how our gut runs when we are aware of and attentive to its natural circadian rhythm, by practicing intermittent fasting and a proper ketogenic diet.

The 12-hour shift in this analogy represents the two separate time frames of our body when properly attuned with our gut's "circadian rhythm". In the real world what this means is the "doors" to our gut open at noon (in our case whenever we first consume something in the morning or early afternoon that is not water). This kickstarts our gut for the day, signaling that it is time to begin the process of taking in food and nutrients for up to the next 12 hours.

The slow opening period would be when we are still fasting but might have our morning ritual of *Naked Coffee* with butter and MCT oil. While still technically fasting at this point, the gut begins the process of turning fat to fuel for the day. When we eventually break our fast, having given our gut plenty of time to prepare, it runs smoothly and efficiently, breaking down the nutrition we take in, providing long term, stabilized energy. A few more hours in between until our final meal of the day and the gut is ready to once again take in and process our fat, and nutrient dense final meal of the day.

Now we've finished the "dinner rush" and ideally our gut will have one to three hours left to begin breaking down the rest of the nutrients and minerals we've taken in through the day. By the time we've reached "closing time" (the end of our 12-hour window), our guts have had more than enough time to process and filter out all the nutrition we've taken in for the day. Now the circadian rhythm is switched to maintenance mode for the next 12-hours, ready and waiting to do the whole thing over again. This is the *ideal* world, but what does reality look like for most of us?

Imagine our same restaurant, with the same hours as before, except this time our workers are called in four hours early to work. They arrive with no time to prep beforehand, and things start to get out of control quickly. The kitchen has had no time to prepare, the restaurant's tables and chairs have not been properly cleaned and reset for the current days' work, yet the staff must trudge on regardless.

Two hours into their early and unprepared start, the staff is hit again. This time a tour bus drops off a group of young children and their chaperones. The restaurant is not prepared for this huge influx of children, and has a daunting lack of high chairs and no kids' menus prepared. The customers, however, have little regard for the restaurant, waitstaff or their *ideal* standards.

They flood in and make crazy demands, ordering things not even offered on the menu. This barrage continues until finally all of the chaperones and children have been served and leave. The aftermath takes loads of time and energy to clean, leaving the staff already flustered and over worked with still another 12 hours left in their day.

Another few hours pass and the normal lunch crowd does not appear. Instead, spurts of people filter in and out the whole day. None of the customers treat the waitstaff well or leave much as far as tips, and again the restaurant staff is deflated as there seems to be no rhyme nor reason to this inconsistent influx of people.

The normal dinner rush begins much later than normal, within 30 minutes of closing time! The restaurant staff is already in the process of shutting things down and now it's as if all the worst types of customers have merged at the doors all at the same time; children en masse and over demanding and rude customers. The restaurant is understaffed at this point and ill-suited to handle the onslaught.

It's already well past midnight and customers still filter in, the normal closing duties cannot be finished and finally around 3 am, the restaurant closes its doors, leaving behind a disaster in its wake, shoddy cleaning, and no prep for tomorrow. Before the staff leaves, they are told, that this is how the restaurant will run for the foreseeable future so everyone should prepare for another day like today, starting bright and early tomorrow morning.

The reality is this second "restaurant" is how most of us treat our gut. Starting in the morning with a full breakfast lacking sufficient nutrients and well before our bodies are even prepared to process it. Assume you wake up at 7 am and eat before work, then after arriving you partake in a donut, or three. You then spend the rest of your work day snacking away on whatever garbage is available to you. Finally, after arriving home you prepare some massive dinner filled with carbohydrates and then follow it up with a dessert, still snacking all the way until you find it's absolutely time for bed; only to repeat the whole thing over again when you wake.

We may not think about it while we're doing it, but this second way of approaching eating is why so many people have a hard time sticking with and succeeding on a diet. Even if our meals are "healthier", we still give our gut too little time to process all the food we eat, and we eat well past the times we should. This is why *when* we eat is just as much, if not more important than *what* we eat.

I hope this analogy was not too conflating or confusing, but rather served to give you an understanding of how we can apply the principles of Intermittent Fasting (with the aid of *Naked Coffee*), a Ketogenic Diet, and our gut's circadian rhythm together to make our diet as efficient and productive as possible. Basically, our diet is three-fold and will look like this:

#1: We eat no more than 12-hours a day, using *Naked Coffee* to assist in longer periods of fasting (*Intermittent Fasting*)

#2: We put at least 12-hours between our last meal of one day and our first meal (or anything other than water) of the next, and we shoot for 9-12 hours *total* of ingesting anything, on any given day (*Gut's Circadian Rhythm*)

#3: We shoot for a high-fat, moderate protein, low-carb diet (*Ketogenics*)

Combining these three ideas together, we can maximize efficiency, and minimize difficulty of retention to this program. We can begin to change the way we think about food and how it works with, and affects, our body. Most importantly, we can start making small changes which can have dramatic impacts on our metabolism and how our bodies react to and process food and nutrition. This is where things really start to come together, and the magic of H.2.L.G.N. starts to turn from a distant mirage, to a realistic achievable program of action.

One last bit on why the Gut's "Circadian Rhythm" is so vital. One of the main studies quoted by Dr. Patrick when discussing this idea was a Harvard rat study. In this study it was found that rats who ate for extended periods throughout the day (longer than 12-hours), increased their risk for numerous diseases, decreased aerobic capacity, increased fat retention, and overall fared poorly. This was true of the rats on a poor diet (high fat & high sugar). Rats on a "healthy" diet didn't see nearly as many detrimental effects, but also didn't receive any beneficial effects.

The rats who maintained a moderately healthy to average diet, but stayed within the 9-10 hours eating window experienced some amazing outcomes. Even without adding exercise, they decreased body fat, and increased lean muscle mass, as well as reducing their risk of developing disease, and increase aerobic capacity. *Without Exercise!*

Purely from limiting their time frame the rats were able to increase lean muscle mass and decrease body fat.

Subjects who stayed within 10-11 hour eating window daily saw some of these results, and those at 11-12 hour eating window basically didn't see any positive or negative gains. This is why this idea of the limiting the "Gut Window" is so, so important. All other things being equal, this is the easiest thing you can change in your diet in the beginning to start making a difference in the way you look and feel.

Adding the 9-12 hour eating time frame (Also called *Time Restricted Feeding*) to my daily routine, has truly been a game changer for me. This is the thing that made it possible to drop those last five pounds that wouldn't quite go, and more importantly to keep them off. Perhaps the best thing about this information is that you don't have to do it every day. There seemed to be no significant difference in results when the rats strictly maintained eating this way for at least five out of seven days in the week. This means, in the beginning specifically, you can still keep your weekends for yourself. That doesn't mean you should necessarily go "crazy" on the weekends, but it also doesn't mean that you shouldn't...

Down the Rabbit Hole: (What your day-to-day eating will look like, and how to start)

In the last section I mentioned a few times that one of the most important things about this process is giving ourselves some room to work. Attempting to make drastic lifestyle changes and completely overhauling the way we've eaten and treated our bodies all at once is a sure fire way to fail. What I do expect from people who actually want to give this thing a shot, is working within a few constraints. Once you start and see that you are doing, quite literally, the *very minimum* and still noticing changes, I believe that will empower you to take the next steps necessary to continue to push the limits of what you can achieve with a little more effort.

In the first couple of weeks while reading this book and preparing to make some changes, I don't expect you to drastically overhaul your diet, but rather simply be more aware of *what* and *when* you are eating. At some point, we do need to set certain boundaries, as there has to be some level of accountability in your daily life.

The following are the "Zones" that you'll progress through as you continue through this lifestyle change. They get progressively more restrictive as you go farther, but realize that the more restrictive each zone is, the less time I expect you to spend in it (at least at first). For example "Zone 1" is not very restrictive and you should be able to meet the requirements for it 7 days a week. "Zone 3" is very restrictive, and as such you're only expected to spend about 3 days a week there, when you finally make it to that point.

When you are ready to really start this journey in changing your eating habits I expect everyone to realistically stay in the "Zone 1" with relative ease and little disruption to how you already feel. The first 3 assignments have been prepping you to make the transition into this zone. This is a great place to start and even doing these things alone will undoubtedly lead to results. However, there is no wiggle room on these basics, these are things you should be doing EVERY day.

As you get more comfortable in your new lifestyle you can progress to the more "restrictive" zones. These are things you should try to incorporate every couple of days at first, maybe even just once a week. As you get more in tune with your eating habits and the way you feel, you will not only desire to incorporate these things more often, you will enjoy doing so. The Zones are as follows:

Zone 1: Mildly Restrictive (7 days a week):

- *Limiting my gut intake (circadian rhythm) to 12 hours or less per day*
- *Fasting for at least 12 hours every day*
- *Including some type of healthy fat in every meal*
- *Limiting sweets and processed foods whenever possible*
- *Never consuming more than 150 grams of net carbs in a day (holidays and special occasions excluded)*
- *Avoiding fast food whenever possible*
- *Minimizing Alcohol Consumption*

Zone 2: Moderately Restrictive (4-7 Days a week after being in Zone 1 for a month)

- *Limiting my gut intake to 10-11 hours a day*

- *Fasting for up to 12+ hours (women) or 16+ hours (men) every day*
- *Limiting my carbohydrate intake at every meal (less than 75 net carbs/day)*
- *Avoiding eating out more than once a day, saving money and more in control of nutrients*
- *Drinking alcoholic beverages (no more than two, no more than twice a week)*

Zone 3: Majorly Restrictive (3-5 days a week after being in Zone 2 for a month)

- *Limiting my gut intake to no more than 9-10 hours a day*
- *Fasting for up to 18+ hours every day*
- *Monitoring carb intake (keeping to less than 50 net carbs/day)*
- *No sweets, no sugar, no "fun" stuff*
- *Keeping a 70/25/5 (fat/protein/carb) ratio throughout the day (keto)*
- *At 2,000 calories per day, this means 150/125/25 grams (fat/protein/carbs)*
- *If that math looks wrong, it's because fats have a higher caloric content (9 calories/gram, compared to 4 calories/gram for protein and carbs)*
- *Preparing my own meals, and portioning appropriately for the week*
- *Completely abstaining from alcoholic beverages*

By the time we get to "Zone 3" you'll have seen massive changes in the way you feel and the way you look. As we continue on this journey we'll start to add brief but intense bouts of exercise one to two times a week to continue to build upon this solid foundation. Remember however, that diet is far and away the most important part of this process. You can't erase a week's worth of slacking with any amount of gym time, especially when we're trying to minimize our effort and maximize our efficiency.

As you progress through these different zones and learn more about yourself and the way your body responds, remember this: All these things have been extremely effective in my diet, even life changing. What I love most about this program is the simplicity. That being said, the *most effective* tool by far that I've found during this journey has been one within "Zone 3", and it's the first on that checklist for a reason.

"Limiting gut intake to no more than 9-10 hours per day" is something I discussed briefly in the last section. The benefits of which seem like one of those "too good to be true" promises. Ever the skeptic I incorporated these ideas, and the results were astonishing. Within two weeks (strictly adhering 3-5 days a week), I lost an additional 10 pounds and almost 3% body fat on my already, newly lean and fit frame. I also experienced no decrease in my strength levels and in the time since incorporating this 9-10 hour window on a semi regular basis, my strength has continued to increase, along with my lean muscle mass.

This 9-10 hour eating window seems to be the key to weight loss and continued muscle growth, when combined with a proper diet and moderate exercise. In fact, it was so effective for weight loss I had to actually stop doing it so frequently (I shoot for less than 11 hours every day, but only a strict 9-10 hours, 2-3 days per week)). I was concerned that after I dipped under 165 lbs for the first time in over a decade, that I might be losing *too much* weight.

I believe firmly that anyone who follows this program and makes it to the point where they can incorporate this technique will see that its results are not the outlier, they are the norm. However, the reason I've laid out the plan the way I have is to slowly get your foot in the door. Some people can jump straight to "Zone 3", but for most people, "Zones 1&2" will serve as a way to transition into this new lifestyle change. Remember, this program is about retention, better to go slowly and stay committed, then too fast and burnout.

Now that we've got eating habits covered, and I believe very realistically as far as the approach, it's time to explore and deconstruct the way we view exercise. In the next section of this book we will be exploring some common misconceptions about what is, and what is not, exercise. Like everything in this book, many of these things are based in personal experience as well as the newest and most exciting ideas in health and fitness. If you have experience with working out in the past, many of the things discussed in the next section will come as a shock to you. It is not my aim to make bold outlandish declarations for the sake of promotion, this doesn't serve me. The things we will be discussing are well understood in the periphery of "mainstream" gym culture. Some of these ideas predate my birth, others have come to light more and more over the past few years and decades.

The point being, I ask that you approach this next section with an open mind. For whatever reason, many people I've talked to over the years will readily admit that they know little to nothing about proper diet and nutrition, the same is not true for exercise. For those of you with prejudices about exactly how and what constitutes exercise, I ask you to hold judgement. Try to forget your lifetime long indoctrination about what exactly exercise is, and what it's supposed to look like. If you've made it this far you've kept an open mind, let's continue on that journey and go deeper down the rabbit hole...

PART III:

EXERCISE

Exercise vs. Recreation

The following article was something written for the clients and friends of the gym I was previously employed with in Minnesota. This is the gym where I learned many of the foundational principles of exercise as I understand them today. After over a decade as a fitness enthusiast and years as a personal trainer and yoga instructor, this was my new understanding of exercise and its purpose. This article will serve as the reference point for the rest of Part III of this book.

"Exercise is a process whereby the body performs work of a demanding nature, in accordance with muscle and joint function, in a clinically controlled environment, within the constraints of safety, meaningfully loading the muscular structures, to inroad their strength levels, to stimulate a growth mechanism, within minimum time." - Ken Hutchins (Renaissance Exercise)

We've been led to believe that everything we do from yoga to mountain climbing constitutes exercise, but this simply is not the case. Exercise as it has been clinically defined above does not include hobbies, sports, or even organized spinning classes; exercise is a precise clinical undertaking. This is not to say that things we enjoy (weight lifting, swimming, etc.) do not have positive physiological benefits on our bodies, but they are not by definition exercise.

These things we do for passion, for pleasure, or even under the misguided assumption of "working out" are in fact recreation. This may seem like a moot point, but the reason it's so important is that it separates what we do at My Strength Studio from what you choose to do for recreation on your own. Exercise should be viewed as something entirely different through the prism of "Cost/Reward". Proper and consistent exercise improves our life and our bodies for all the other things we enjoy doing in life, but exercise as it has been defined should almost never be "enjoyed" in the traditional sense of the word. We may enjoy the results is gives us, we may enjoy changes to our bodies, but the actual practice of exercise should be viewed more like a clinical undertaking.

Part of staying healthy is eating a diverse diet, getting adequate amounts of sleep, and doing proper and continuous exercise in a controlled and safe environment. This is why at My Strength Studio we have created a system for exercise which fulfills all the clinical requirements, maximizes efficiency, and minimizes the time required. If you do nothing else for your body, spend 20 minutes once or twice a week with us and reap all the benefits of positive enhancements from muscle growth, cardiovascular strengthening, and increased metabolism. If, however, you do have other hobbies, consider adding My Strength Studio to your current training regimen and experience a happier, healthier you, in all the recreational activities you already enjoy.

Ask our clients about how this workout is different from anything they've done before, and for many it is the first "real exercise" of their life. If you're not convinced, come in for a free consult and demo workout and see for yourself what makes My Strength Studio the best, most efficient workout in the country.

Your Pal in Fitness,

Logan Herlihy

(Published February 2018)

So where does this leave us with exercise and how we should approach it from here on out? I made a few bold promises and claims in the beginning of this book and for good reason. Before we get too far into my discovery of "less is more" I want to give you an idea of how I came to arrive at this understanding. It's something that I still struggle with, and for myself, after so many years of being a five-times-a-week gym person, it's incredibly hard to shake those practices.

The truth is I sometimes feel as if I'm not doing enough, because I really do *only workout* 1-2 times per week now (usually only once every 7-10 days), but the results don't lie. Knowing what I know now, and seeing how easy it's been to get in, and more importantly maintain, the best shape of my life, I can't fight it any longer. I was indoctrinated for the better part of a decade to believe that what I was doing was exercise, and it was the only way to achieve my goals. I would have fought people tooth and nail to defend those beliefs.

Now that I have seen the light, it does not change the fact that I was deeply invested in my old thinking for a long time, and old thinking is hard to change. The most frustrating part is I still see people ALL THE TIME doing the same things I used to do, and it's damn near impossible to convert them. Look, if you are proud to be a gym rat and that is part of your personality and what defines you, good for you, there's nothing wrong with that. I'm not so brazen to say that there's anything wrong with devoting your life to two hours at the gym a day, five days a week.

We live in a country where the obesity rate is climbing at pandemic proportions, so to me that is much better than the alternative. What I will say to anyone currently doing that, or that thinks spending endless hours busting ass in the gym is the only way to build an ideal physique... you're wrong.

The vast majority of us will never be bodybuilders or fitness models, we simply want to look good, be healthy and be comfortable in our own skin (naked perhaps?). You can look good, and more importantly, feel fantastic, simply by exercising *properly* 1-2 times per week for 40 minutes or less (Eventually we will get to 20 minute workouts, but there is an initial "learning curve associated with this type of training that takes some time).

So How Did I Get Here?

When I began my fitness journey over a decade ago, I was a scraggly six-foot, 135-pound, 17-year old going into my senior year of high school. I had always followed my dad around the gym when he would go, but I never really knew what I was doing, and I mostly just screwed around. I was decently athletic, but I was much too skinny to ever actually compete in big time contact sports, running was much more my thing. That year I had had it. I decided I was going to do whatever it took to get big and ripped like my other friends who had been football studs and hit their growth spurts, and puberty long before me.

I bought a gym membership to a local Gold's Gym™ and started going every day. I didn't really know what I was doing at first, but I met some extremely nice (extremely buff) gym rats along the way who helped me on my journey. I was inundated with "bro-science," weight gainer protein powders, creatine, and supplements galore. I even went so far as to cycle on to some over the counter test booster (but I started getting bacne and freaked out).

Within about six months of daily dedication, constant research and non-stop shoving my face full of protein, I went into my final semester of senior year a bulky, but built 195-pounds of man meat... I had arrived. From that point on for about the next 5-7 years I was purely team "Meathead." I wanted to get bigger, then lean, then bigger again, it consumed me. About five years ago, my mindset started to shift, I realized I was getting stretch marks from bulking and cutting, and I knew I would never compete in lifting so I had a "what's the point?" moment. I decided it would make sense to cut some weight.

I started doing yoga, lifting lighter, trying to do all the things I had forever been told would give me longer, leaner muscles. After losing a little weight I found to my dismay that simply changing my routine wasn't enough, I could never get quite as lean and cut as I wanted. I started a vicious cycle of long intense workouts, followed by longer even more intense bouts of cardio. Again, I lost a little more weight, but it never stayed off and even though I wasn't as big as I used to be, my weight would still fluctuate like crazy. It wasn't uncommon for me to weigh 180 one week and 190 the next, with what I thought had been little to no modification in my lifestyle or routine. I was officially stuck. Flash forward about a year and a half ago, I had started a new job with a new company, and suddenly... everything changed.

To try to fit everything I learned about exercise and nutrition that challenged the status quo would be ill-advised in a book I'm *trying* to make short(ish) and succinct. I can however, give you a rundown of the basics, and begin to introduce some of the ideas and concepts that planted the seeds that eventually blossomed into the book you hold in your hands today. The article in the beginning of this section is a broad overview of something I practice in my work and personal life. Here's the long and the short of it.

In the 1980's there was a revolutionary fitness mind who was one of the original developers of Nautilus Equipment. His name is Dr. Ken Hutchins. Dr. Hutchins was obsessed from a young age with the human form and its strength potential. (He also really likes to compare bodies and training to playing the Trumpet... which he will constantly tell you he was fantastic at!) Through his research and development with Nautilus, you could argue that Dr. Hutchins became obsessed with the idea of how to maximize humans' strength and physical form potential. At some point in his research he was commissioned to develop a study for the University of Florida, tracking the effects of low impact strength training on Osteoporosis in the elderly female population (I promise there's a point here).

Through his research (some would say by accident) he stumbled upon a method for exercise, strength training specifically, the results of which were beyond his wildest dreams. He found by working extremely intensely, but also going through movements extremely slowly, his patients experienced not only a decrease in signs of osteoporosis, but a slew of other physiological and metabolic benefits. Through this study, an idea was borne which eventually developed into a modality called *SuperSlow*™, which has since spawned dozens of variations and derivations over the decades. Now, I tell you all of that to explain the following. Without diving too deeply into the exact metabolic and physiological reasons for why this training style is so effective, it helps to think about the general overview of the ideas like this.

#1: *The most important part of the human physiology is the human muscular skeletal structure.* If you increase the muscles' ability to function optimally and efficiently, you in turn increase the rest of the body's ability to function optimally and efficiently. (The important part here is that everything trickles down, starting with the muscles, the inverse of this is not true).

An example of this would be that by increasing the muscular functionality of the body, you as a result, naturally increase cardiovascular capacity. You cannot however, attempt to increase cardiovascular capacity in hopes of increasing muscular functionality.

#2: *The greater the stimulus, the greater the resulting change.* However, this is a process of diminishing returns. Meaning you cannot expect to create the same stimulus every time and get the same results. As the change or degree of adaptation increases, so must the ensuing stimulus.

Without trying to get too scientific that means if a stimulus (S = 1) creates an adaptation (A =1), the first time, the adaptation will be slightly diminished the next time you apply the same stimulus.

Week 1 of Workout S1 = A1

Week 2 of Workout S1 = A0.9

Week 3 of Workout S1 = A0.8

Etc., Etc., on to infinity

An easy analogy for this is getting a tan. If you stay out in the sun for 30 minutes and get burned, your body adapts by making you tan. This way the next time you're out in the sun you won't get burned by the same time in the sun. If you want to keep tanning, you have to keep increasing the stimulus (time in the sun) to keep getting an adaptation (darker tan). So exactly what the hell does all that mean? What that means and how Dr. Hutchins applied it is this: *If you push your body to its limit in a short, intense bout of exercise (20-40 minutes) you will initiate a natural adaptive response.* This adaption will ensure that you are more prepared to handle these same forces the next time you encounter them. So even though we are only exercising 1-2 times per week, when we exercise, we are working so intensely that our bodies (forced into a state of literal "fight or flight") are forced to physically adapt due to the stimulus.

Sufficient Stimulus —> Physical Adaptation

This is a very different approach to exercise than the casual approach we are constantly bombarded with through modern gyms and fitness advertisements. It even varies from the more intense bodybuilder mentality you see worshipped in documentaries like "Pumping Iron". When we exercise, we want to deliberately force ourselves to the point that our Darwinian response kicks in telling us, *"Adapt or Die!"*. When I started at My Strength Studio my boss explained it to me this way.

"Logan, imagine you are living in the hunter-gatherer times. As you are out collecting food you get attacked out of nowhere by a mountain lion. You manage to wrestle with it and fight it off, but it comes close to taking your life. From an evolutionary perspective your body has just experienced an incredibly traumatizing stimulus. However, being the extremely adaptive creatures we are, your body adapts to this stimulus making you stronger and more physically imposing, so the next time you will be better suited for a

similar circumstance. *That's essentially what we are trying to do here, prepare you to fight the mountain lion."*

-      *Kevin Ness, Owner of My Strength Studio*

Let's just say that was an intense first day (Jesus Kevin! I thought we were just doing freaking leg press!). But he was right, and that's the attitude I've carried into my exercise routine from that day on. In doing so, I get the advantage of working out much less frequently than I used to, and by always increasing the stimulus (in this case, the weights) I'm able to constantly improve and get ready to face the proverbial "mountain lion".

Exercise *or* Recreation

We'll get more into how you're going to get started into this new idea of exercise (what workouts will look like, where you should workout, etc.) a little later, but let's talk a little more about the difference between these two ideas. While many people I talk to have no experience with exercise and are excited about the idea of only one to two sessions a week, there are also quite a few who seem discouraged about not working out as much. Some people (myself included) really enjoy going to the gym. I need to make a few things clear for the purpose of being completely transparent.

I still go to the gym when I can, but I don't count those visits as "exercise". Like I said I've been a 5-7 times a week gym guy for the better part of a decade. I could say old habits are hard to break, but the truth is I just like being at the gym. What's changed the most with my "recreational" visits throughout the week is they in no way constitute exercise as we have now defined it. When I go to the gym now I might do some yoga, hit the heavy bag, do some crunches, but mostly I'm just there because I like the environment (and the sauna).

The reason I'm telling you this is because I would be a hypocrite if I said you should never do anything except your one to two exercise routines a week. You don't have to, but you can, and sometimes I choose to, because I like being active. When my schedule has been too crazy I often can't make my extra weekly "recreational" gym visits. The truth is these visits probably only serve to delay my recovery and prevent me from adapting for my following *actual exercise* visit. The reason I'm telling you all this is because if you do yoga three days a week, you are a runner, or you just enjoy lifting casually, you can still do all of those things. The important part here is you don't *have to* you *get to.*

Having recreational fitness hobbies is a great thing, fantastic even. But what I want is for this book to be all inclusive. For everyone who tries this program that is currently doing little to no physical activity, there might be another person who wants to take the next step in their fitness journey, but isn't quite ready to give up on Pilates, CrossFit, or whatever the hell else they're doing.

I just want you to know that H.2.L.G.N. is an all-inclusive group. I'm going to give you the tools to do the absolute *least amount* possible to get great results, if that's all you're after great! If that's just the tip of the iceberg and you want to smash a CrossFit competition or run a marathon, there's room enough for all of us... so let's get started!

Assumed vs. Real Objective

If you look in any magazine, see any ads on T.V. or have ever had a consult with a personal trainer at most major gyms then you're already aware of a major problem with most exercise regimens. Most training programs, magazines, books, etc. focus on something in training called the "Assumed Objective".

The Assumed Objective is essentially a metrics, or quantitative based way of approaching fitness. Think 3 sets of 10 reps of 25 lbs. As you gain strength and continue along the progression of your program, you increase your metrics, and in doing so, increase your strength and gains. While this makes logical sense, when you focus purely on metrics, you lose sight of what's actually important when we approach exercise from a more clinical perspective.

Essentially, what we are attempting to do through exercise is create a stimulus message powerful enough to produce a physiological adaptation in your body. Metrics are of little to no importance as far as your body is concerned. What is important, is the severity and the quality of the stimulus. This is why many people who approach programs from a metrics standpoint X amount of sets, with Y amount of reps, with Z amount of weight, end up stagnating. The amount of stimulus your body needs from day-to-day can vary greatly based on a variety of factors including, mood, sleep, energy, etc. So to assume the theory of applying a consistent metric based program you will achieve a maximum stimulus each and every time you exercise is just ill-conceived.

Let's look at a different analogy to help explain this idea in a little more detail. Assume you're studying for an upcoming exam in let's say,

World History. The way most exercise programs approach this exam is to focus exclusively on American History. You study for 2-hours a day, 5-days a week, but you only cover this one topic. You will most likely get *really* good at American History, but you will be ill-served when exam time comes and all you've done is focus all your time and attention on a quantitative understanding of just *one topic* of History, American History, instead of World History.

Instead what we will be focusing on with the exercise approach outlined in this book is the "Real Objective". The real objective in exercise is to approach and move past the point of Inroad (the momentary weakening or fatiguing of the muscles) each and every time we exercise. Though metrics are a part of this equation, we are more concerned with the quality of the work, as a opposed to the quantity.

Instead of measuring each exercise in reps, sets, and weights, we are instead focused on getting to something called Momentary Muscle Failure (or MMF). MMF is the point during the exercise when you can no longer continue through a rep with good form, and you've literally failed in that moment. By measuring the effectiveness of our workouts this way, we can assure that we are creating an effective stimulus each and every time we work out, significant enough to cause a physiological adaptation in our bodies.

Assumed Objective:
- Quantitative Approach
- Increase Metrics (sets, reps, weights, etc.)
- Goal to make all metrics go UP

Real Objective:
- Qualitative Approach
- Achieve Inroad/MMF every time
- Goal: Stimulus -> Body -> Adaptation

Stimulus→ Response:

The easiest example for many people to understand how our bodies adapt to an outside stimulus is thinking of going out in the sun. If you're like me (super white and pasty) the unprotected sun presents my body with a stimulus, which creates an physical adaptation (I turn red, then hopefully tan). Assuming I continue to apply a similar stimulus, my body (now tan) will not continue to change unless I continually increase the intensity of the stimulus (sun exposure). This is similar to how we want to approach exercise. Once an adaptation has been achieved (we are stronger), we must continue to increase the severity of the stimulus each time to achieve a greater and greater adaptation.

Using our studying analogy again, this qualitative approach would be the equivalent of not just studying, but learning a new and different part of World History each and every time we sit down. Some days this might equate to a few hours of learning and grasping new concepts foreign to us, others we might gain all the information we need in just 30 minutes. In this scenario we are focused on the actual quality of the studying and the knowledge gained as opposed to simply studying the same material over and over, just for the sake of studying.

To achieve the Real Objective each and every time we exercise we are going to need to follow certain guidelines. The following graph describes the course of exercise in the H.2.L.G.N. method versus traditional exercise at the gym.

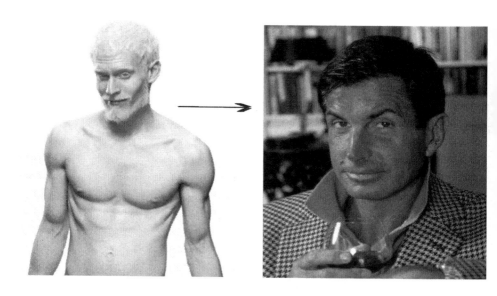

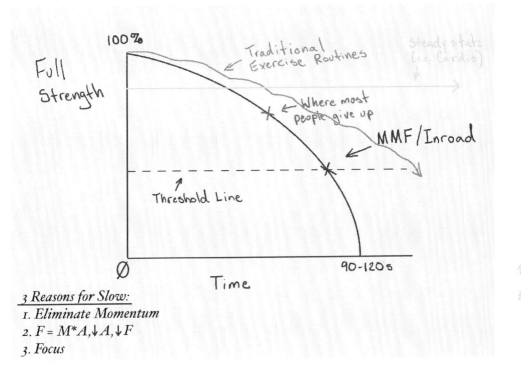

100%

Full
Strength

Traditional
Exercise Routines

Steady state
(in Cardio)

Where most
people give up

MMF/Inroad

Threshold Line

Ø

Time

90-120s

3 Reasons for Slow:
1. Eliminate Momentum
2. F = M*A, ↓A, ↓F
3. Focus

3 Reasons for Moving Slowly:

The reason we want to move slowly (4-12 seconds in both the positive and negative direction of each lift) is three-fold. The first reason is to eliminate momentum. In most gyms you will see people moving through repetitions extremely quickly. By creating momentum in swinging their joints, they allow themselves to complete more repetitions, but the actual muscle does little to no work as momentum takes over for the majority of the movement. When you move slowly, no momentum is created.

The second reason is to decrease force. When you decrease your momentum that's another way of saying a decrease in acceleration through a movement. For anyone that's ever taken a Physics class you will remember that F(force)= M(mass)*A(acceleration). If you decrease the acceleration of a movement, then you in turn decrease the overall force. This is extremely important for safety as there can be a drastic difference in the force output between a "normal" quick repetition, and moving 4-12 seconds in each direction.

Finally, moving slowly allows us to focus on our repetitions in a way that moving quickly through them does not. When your reps take 4-12 seconds in either direction, you feel everything going on at a deep physiological level in your muscles. This becomes increasingly more important as we learn the difference between discomfort and actual failure. Most people moving quickly don't understand this difference and simply give up on a set either at, or well before failure, usually when they become uncomfortable.

Understanding the reasons for moving slowly and approaching MMF and maximum Inroad each and every time we exercise, will now prepare us even more for this undertaking. In the next section we will be discussing something called the "Time/Intensity Principle", before finally getting started with the actual format of the protocol. All these ideas, just like with our dieting, continue to build on each other, and together will make for the most effective and time efficient workouts possible.

Time/Intensity Principle

Before we even dive into this idea which makes the workout principles explained in the last section of this book applicable to the real world, I feel like I need to once again approach this subject with caution. There are a number of well more qualified and more educated proponents of this modality who can explain in such depth, and detail that I stand in awe. One of these experts is a gentleman named Dr. Doug McGuff who took Dr. Hutchins' ideas and has expounded on them beautifully. He wrote a book called "Body by Science" which is arguably the most informative and approachable book when dealing with this specific modality, which at first can be hard to believe. I would recommend reading *Body by Science* to anyone who desires a deeper understanding of the physiological principles involved in this modality.

Though Dr. McGuff does a fantastic job of delving deeper into these subjects, he is still long winded to some extent in his explanations. What I am attempting to do in this book is take these highly complex and scientifically detailed ideas, and package them in a way that is approachable. For anyone so inclined, you can use this as a springboard to dive as deeply down into this topic as you would like. At the same time I don't want to discriminate against those who simply are looking for the fundamentals of this program to apply efficiently and easily into their own daily lives.

INVERSE RELATIONSHIP: TIME/INTENSITY

At the core of the exercise modality I'm advocating in this program is a principle about the inverse relationship between time and intensity when working out. This relationship is essentially the following:

As Time (T) of Exercise Increases, available Intensity (I) for Exercise Decreases: If T↑, then I↓

As Intensity (I) of Exercise Increases, available Time (T) for Exercise Decreases: If I↑, the T↓

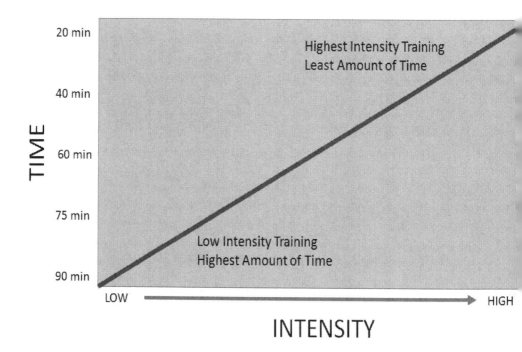

This is an idea we all inherently know, but is not often talked about in modern health and fitness. The idea being that the more time you have for exercise, the less intense that exercise must be, and vice versa. The more intense the exercise, the less time the exercise will be. Think about it in the terms of a race. In a marathon, for example, you would not go at 100 percent effort right from the starting line, you would instead pace yourself to ensure you had enough intensity (or effort) to last for the entire race (If T↑, then I↓). On the other hand, if you were participating in a 100-meter dash you would see no use in saving energy, but rather would go with a maximum effort from the start. But, immediately upon finishing the sprint you would be entirely sapped of energy because your intensity was so much higher (If I↑, then T↓).

This idea has become extremely popular in the last decade with a new type of training under the banner of H.I.I.T. (High Intensity Interval Training). If you ever been to an Orangetheory Fitness, or a CrossFit gym, or anywhere else that promotes a great workout in "1-Hour or Less!", they are under the umbrella of H.I.I.T. Though these ideas may be rooted in similar principles, these gyms and workout styles still vary greatly from what we are attempting to do in H.2.L.G.N. An hour is still far too long for our purposes.

With the *SuperSlow*™ method developed by Dr. Hutchins, and the vast improvements made by Dr. McGuff, what we will be doing is more like H.I.T. (High Intensity Training). The removal of that second "I" representing the "Interval" is something that will become increasingly more important as we go farther down this path. H.I.I.T. training is like lightly jogging around a 400m track and "sprinting" the corners. What we going to be doing is all out sprinting in a 100m dash... in slow-motion. This is where things start to get interesting.

The Protocol: Part I

(Where are we doing this?)

In the ideal world we would be partaking in this type of training method in a gym equipped with *SuperSlow™, MedEx™, or Nautilus™* designed equipment... alas, we do not live in an ideal world. I'm fortunate in my field to work in places where I have all these machines available to me. In this next section we are going to discuss what a workout will look like if you don't currently have access to a state-of-the-art training facility.

Though having this exact type of equipment can potentially take our training to the next level, for the purposes of this book, any gym will do. As long as your gym meets the following criteria, you should have everything you need to get the most from your workouts.

#1: *Equipment from the last decade*: though there are some gyms that maintain high quality, older equipment, for the most part if your gym has really old equipment it's probably ill-maintained.

#2: *A time that's not completely packed during the day*: it's great to be able to socialize at the gym, but not for the purposes of what we're doing. Finding a time with minimum people around while not necessary, will definitely make the process of exercise, easier and more efficient.

Those two simple criteria should allow you to follow this program about as well as one could hope for. I don't expect anyone to go out and spend $100/month on a gym membership, especially if you're only going there 1-2 times per week. There are SO many gyms available these days, *Anytime Fitness™, Planet Fitness™, LA Fitness™,* even your local

YMCA™. There are modifications that can be made for body-weight exercises you can do at home or on the road, but you really should have a gym membership by the time you're ready to start the exercise portion of this program, and you should be able to find something for a decent price (Groupon has lots of deals).

The Protocol: Part II

(What is it, and how does it work?)

Once again, we find ourselves in a predicament. I'm going to attempt to explain some extremely complex ideas in a way that doesn't go on ad nauseum. Just like with every other part of this book however, I encourage anyone who wishes to dive deeper into this subject to do just that. Both Dr. Hutchins and Dr. McGuff have written extensive volumes on what I am about to attempt to sum up in the next few pages.

If you simply want to take me at my word and get this thing started as quickly as possible, go for it! However, if you do find this information extremely revolutionary and interesting the way I did, then go forward and explore! There is a massive amount of data to get lost under. That being said, let's give this a try...

The prevailing knowledge about exercise has basically dumbed down the actual science and physiology behind exactly *what* exercise is supposed to accomplish, and *why*, when properly applied it can do just that. If we were to define the actual purpose of exercise, I believe it might look something like this.

Exercise Purpose: *to improve the strength and functionality of the muscular skeletal structure of the human body and its reciprocal components (i.e. heart, lungs, digestive system, etc.) to maximize the body's ability to deal with both seen and unforeseen obstacles within the environment.*

When we look at this version of the purpose of exercise it drastically changes the way we will go on viewing traditional ideas about exercise. When your *primary purpose* is to improve the muscular skeletal structure, a lot of other programs considered by some to be "exercise" begin to fall away. The only way to improve the muscular skeletal structure is through strength training, and the most effective and efficient way to do that is with structured, safe, and intense training sessions. In a traditional strength training workout, you might expect to see repetitions taking less than a second each way on both the concentric and eccentric parts of a movement (up and down). With the Bicep Curl, for instance, it's not uncommon to see someone get 20 reps on alternating curls on both arms in a minute or less.

While this might make us feel good that we've moved a certain amount of weight a certain amount of times, in actuality this serves little to no purpose as far as muscle growth and increased strength. What we're trying to accomplish through exercise is a stimulus powerful enough to trigger growth and change. Flying through repetitions will never accomplish this. Instead with the H.2.L.G.N. exercise program, what we are going to attempt in our workouts is getting to Momentary Muscle Failure (MMF). The way we do this is four-fold in our workouts.

#1: *Repetitions should take 4-12 seconds on both the positive and negative portions of the exercise (10 seconds being the ideal, but not the requirement).*

#2: *Eliminating rest throughout the course of the movement by never fully unloading the muscles.*

#3: *Capping our repetitions for a given exercise at 20 total (depending on speed of motion) and trying to stay within a highly defined minimum/maximum window of time (90-180 seconds) referred to as Time Under Load (T.U.L.).*

#4: *Tracking and logging all exercises including Date, Exercise, Weight, Reps, Total TUL, and Average Rep Speed in order to constantly push forward and make improvements in each and every workout.*

Let's take some time to review each of these ideas a little more in-depth to see why each is an important and vital step, and how they work together in unison to give us the most effective workout in the least amount of time. The reason we are moving in 4-12 seconds (in each direction) is to properly stimulate all the muscles in a given exercise because of the difference in muscle fibers and their efficiency. Let's go back to our Bicep Curl example from earlier (with sub one second positives and negatives) and explore the differences between this type of workout and what we are going to be doing with H.2.L.G.N.

In the previous example with the fast-moving curls, the muscle fibers in the arms aren't under load long enough for the arms to actually fatigue towards failure, instead your arms simply become tired from overuse. However, when we slow down the repetition sequence to 4-12 seconds in either direction, the varying muscle fibers in the arms begin to break down throughout the course of the repetitions. As we continue to stay slow and move continuously through the reps the second level fibers in the arms are recruited in order to give the first fibers a brief recovery period. *If you were to just stop here and set the bar down, within moments your first level fibers would become almost completely recovered, this is why it's so important to make sure we never fully unload during the course of a set. In order to make sure we break down all the appropriate fibers, we must keep our muscles under consistent tension throughout the entire repetition cycle.* When that recovery period does not come however, the fibers continue to fatigue, switching back and forth between themselves, each one trying to give the other some much-needed rest.

Finally, when they have quite literally nothing left to give you will find that no matter how hard you try, you cannot move another inch. In

111

this moment you have reached Momentary Muscle Failure. You should still continue to struggle with the weight here (even though it will no longer be moving) for another 5-10s. Only then should you slowly set the weight down and move on to the next exercise, to repeat the whole process over again.

That explanation takes care of the first two parts of the workout, as the entire point of this exercise program is to create maximum stimulus within minimal time. With a 5-7 exercise movement routine, and a maximum of three minutes per exercise, there is no reason you shouldn't be able to accomplish a completely devastating workout in under 40 minutes (and much less as you get more efficient moving from machine to machine, and your weights get more and more challenging). The last two parts of the equation (capping at 20 reps and maintaining detailed notes) become exceedingly more important the farther along we get into this program. This brings us to the final part of our protocol.

The Protocol: Part III

(What are we doing?)

There is a steep learning curve with this particular type of training. Most of us are not used to pushing our bodies to the limits they will be forced to in H.I.T. This is why in the initial phases of our training (as we figure out our ideal weights and familiarize ourselves with *how exactly* to do these workouts) the 20-rep or 180-second (3-minute) caps are so important (Step 3). If we start off with too light of a weight on a particular exercise, we may be able to continue (even at such a slow speed) for drastically too long. Not necessarily risking injury, but more so boredom and wasted time. This is where Step 4 (*Tracking and logging all exercises*) becomes especially important.

Taking detailed notes each time we exercise will help us to faster approach our goals of staying in that 20-rep and 180-second cap limit. If a weight is too light when we first attempt it and we make it to three minutes barely fatigued, we know that next time we will need to increase our weight on that exercise to fall within that time window and work towards M.M.F. On the other hand, if we attempt a weight on a certain exercise and find we cannot make it to the minimum of 90-seconds, we know we have overshot the mark. Next time we should ratchet the weight down a bit and see if we now fall into that window with our failure.

When we break down what exercises we will be doing later in this section we will go a little farther into some general starting guidelines for men and women with regards to weights. Just remember there is no rush, take your time and be nice to your body. If you are following the dietary restrictions outlined earlier in this book, the exercise will just be serving as an added bonus for weight loss and overall health and wellness goals. There are no prizes for getting your weights exactly right the first time and conservative estimates for adjusting weights are as follows.

If you find a weight is much too light when starting out, ratchet it up by 5% for the next workout and try again until you find yourself within the appropriate window. If you find you cannot manage even the minimum T.U.L. with a certain weight, bring it down 15-20% for the next workout and attempt to find yourself within the appropriate window. On a personal note, I have fine-tuned my weights to the point where I will rarely spend more than 120 seconds on any one exercise, while making sure I maintain my appropriate 4-12 seconds in each direction. This means, each exercise I do rarely lasts more than 10 total repetitions (almost always 6-8 total reps *max* on each exercise).

Some people prefer longer time under loads, some people wish to be done as quickly as humanly possible, the only one who knows what you prefer is you. Experiment, using your detailed notes as a way to push the limits of your T.U.L. and rep counts. There are an endless variety of ways to get completely obliterated doing this workout within the defined time frame, the choice is yours.

The entire premise of this program is "The Least Amount of Effort", and that's true, to an extent. If you follow the H.2.L.G.N. exercise program to a "T" you will certainly be doing *less* exercise than you would in other programs, but don't mistake that with *easy*, because easy it is not. The thing that makes this program so effective and efficient, is because though we exercise infrequently, when we do exercise, we do so with maximum intensity. In order to do this properly and with the most effectiveness there are a few things that we must understand about this training program. This only works if we continue to challenge our bodies, and the best way to continuously challenge ourselves is to know what we've accomplished in the past. Charting progress is a vital step in this protocol, as this will allow us to make sure we are always pushing ourselves further, and continuing to get stronger.

There are only five foundational exercise movements in this program (with a multitude of other additional movements available), but for the purposes of starting out, we are only worried about those five. By keeping track of our routine in real time from workout to workout we can gauge progress from each previous workout. As we get farther along even if our weights do not go up from a previous workout, we may still be able to increase our "Time Under Load".

The Workouts

(20-40 Minutes, 1-2 X per week)

We've made it to the exciting part! Now we actually get to see what types of exercises we'll be doing and what our weekly workouts will actually look like. Let me just say congrats on getting this far and really committing to understanding the *Why* before we actually get into the *How*. Without truly understanding the principles of this modality you would be ill-prepared to start this exercise protocol. By understanding *Why* we're doing what we're doing, you will have a much better appreciation of the *How* we are doing it.

Unlike traditional exercise routines, the learning curve for H.I.T. training is extremely high. You cannot expect to show up on the gym on Day 1 and just "Get it". For the purposes of this training you really need to "feel it", and that takes some time. With a properly educated trainer, in a facility with high-tech training equipment, we can expect that the typical learning curve of a new client training two times per week to start will be approximately 4-8 weeks. Since we don't know what type of equipment you will have available, and you will be doing this on your own, I would conservatively estimate this process taking 8-12 weeks before you really start to *feel* what we're doing here.

This doesn't mean that you will be busting your ass in the gym 2-3 times a week for 2-3 months to start. In fact, quite the opposite. In this beginning phase give yourself a little more time (upwards of 40-60 minutes) when you go to the gym. These sessions shouldn't be too physically taxing. Your first few sessions specifically, you will need to identify the appropriate equipment (where is it in the gym), and begin to hone in your weights, as well as formulating what your routines will look like. After about 2-4 weeks of laying the groundwork, you should be ready to start going through your workouts with a little more efficiency (maybe 30-45 minutes in the gym).

These next 2-4 weeks you should continue to get more comfortable with the routines and hone in your weights to the most appropriate levels. You should really start focusing on your form and making minor improvements in it each time you exercise (As a general rule, you shouldn't be very far under the 180-second cap during this period, this is the opportunity to very slowly increase weights and perfect position before the workouts become incredibly physically demanding).

The final 2-6 weeks of this initial discovery period will be a process of you getting increasingly more efficient with your routine (20-40 minutes). This means your weights are starting to get more challenging, your form is staying consistent, and you're starting to get to the point of Momentary Muscle Failure by the end of your workout. These sessions will start moving quicker and you will begin to start feeling that you are needing more recovery time in between your workouts. The whole process should breakdown something like this:

-       ***Phase I*** *(Groundwork):* Weeks 1-4 going to the gym. In this phase you're identifying equipment needed, getting acclimated to the style, and building your planning and charting for your workouts going forward. Workouts should be little to low-difficulty. *(2-3 sessions/week, 40-60 minutes)*

- **Phase II** *(Getting Acclimated):* Weeks 2-6 going to the gym. In this phase you should feel much more comfortable with the process of your charting, and your workout. You're going through full workouts at this point, but more concerned with correcting form discrepancies, and dialing in appropriate weights. Workouts should be low-difficulty, and not reaching failure. *(2-3 sessions/week, 30-45 minutes)*

- **Phase III** *(Improving Efficiency):* Weeks 7-12 going to the gym. In this phase you should be extremely comfortable with your routine. You won't be getting to MMF most of the time, but you will be flirting with it as you continue to increase your weights and your efficiency. You'll start to notice that you feel the need for longer periods of recovery, and you're ready to scale back frequency, and scale up intensity. Workouts should be intermediate-moderate difficulty, occasionally getting close to failure. *(1-2 sessions/week, 20-40 minutes)*

- **Phase IV** *(Up and running):* After the initial onboarding and getting up to speed in 8-12 weeks, you should be fully in the swing of things. You should have your routine down to a science at this point, and know what you're going to do that day before you ever step foot in the gym. Your charting should be efficient and comprehensive and you should get to, or close to Momentary Muscle Failure each and every session. From here, constant incremental improvements are the goal, and since your intensity is now ramped up to 100% each and every session, your frequency has been ramped down to only as often as necessary. *(1-2 sessions/week, 20-30 minutes)*

The Big 5 (& Big 7)

Each session should be comprised of main functional muscle groups in the body. Unlike bodybuilding or other types of training styles, there are no isolation training exercises for our purposes. We're trying to accomplish as much as possible, as quickly as possible. This means no Isolation Curls, or Brazilian Butt Lifts, instead we'll be focusing on large compound movements, that utilize as many muscle groups as possible with each lift. In the beginning it might seem by doing this that we are failing to maximize certain ideal body parts (Abs, Triceps, Biceps, etc.). As we continue to improve in our efficiency and our weights constantly increase, you will quickly begin to notice how each compound movement more than sufficiently targets all these focus areas we may have.

The main foundational workout of H.2.L.G.N. consists of only five compound movements. They are as follows:

H.2.L.G.N. "Big 5" Workout Routine

1. Leg Press
2. Seated Supinated Grip Pull-down
3. Seated Chest Press
4. Seated Parallel Grip Compound Row
5. Seated Overhead Press

In an ideal world, those five exercises listed above will be all you have to do, 1-2 times per week to maintain peak physical condition. There is an endless variety of ways to mix up this workout to suit your individual needs, but at its root, this entire program boils down to those five exercises. This is also why it's so important to understand and explain the reasoning and science behind this specific type of method before simply showing you those exercises. Without knowing the process and the precise nature in which we are going to perform those movements, one may glance at those five exercises and think,

"That's it?! That's freaking it? That's what you spent the last 50 plus pages leading up to was leg press and chest press?! Well duh! No shit Sherlock!"

Again, the basis of this whole modality is simplicity and efficiency. It then makes sense that the most fundamental exercises, when tweaked to our specific requirements, have the capacity to be the most devastating and most efficient exercises available. In addition to the "Big 5", there are a few other exercises we can add in to accommodate some additional strength gains, and what we're going to explore next is what your starting routine should look like in your first few sessions in the gym.

The charting for your first session and future sessions should look something like the following:

Workout #1	Seat/Settings	Notes	(Date of Workout)
(Machine Type) Exercise [sequence #]	Seat 2, Seatback3	Injuries, ROM, etc.	Weight/Reps (Time)
(Hammer Strength) Seated Calf Raise [1]	N/A	Watch stretch at bottom ROM	100/10 (120)
(Nautilus) Trunk Extension [2]	Seat 2, Pad 3	Limited ROM at bottom, progress slowly	90/8 (115)
(Hammer Strength) Leg Press [3]	Seat 5, Back 3	Left Knee issue, stop reps at 10	250/9 (150)
(Life Fitness) Pulldown [4]	Seat4, Neutral Grip bar	Rotating Neutral and Supinated grip	120/14 (140)

(Cybex) Horizontal Handle Chest Press [5]	Seat 3	Watch shoulder impingement at bottom	140/10 (90)
(Hammer Strength) Seated Row [6]	Seat 2	N/A	120/8 (140)
(Cybex) Overhead Press [7]	Seat 3, Pad 2	Watch shoulder impingement at bottom	80/10 (120)
Exercise Notes:			

As you can see from this example chart, this format has all the space you will need to chart and track your progress for future workouts. The highlighted portions represent the purpose of each column and what it should be used for. For example in the "Notes" column you should be recording any injuries, range of motion issues, or just notes about each particular exercise movement you feel are important. This chart is easily replicable on a program like Google Sheets, and whether you use paper or digital, I would highly recommend you keep detailed records as you make progress through this program.

This is where you will track all your different exercise movements, starting with the "Big 5" and adding and subtracting different exercises as you see fit throughout the course of your training. You'll notice in the example above, I have two additional exercises (calf raise and trunk extension). All you will need to get started is the "Big 5", but you have the option to add on to that as you advance through training.

All supplemental exercise movements will be outlined in the "Appendix" section at the end of the book. For most people the "Big 5" will be the easiest and most appropriate starting point for any new exercise routine, but consult the Appendix for any modifications you may need either starting out, or as you progress further through the protocol.

With each new workout, you can simply copy and paste your chart from the previous workout and change the machines (if different) and the weights accordingly, as you progress through that particular workout. Make sure you are also noting the "Workout #" and the date of that particular workout. This is an invaluable tool when tracking progress, especially as you continue to increase your strength throughout the program. When we see how quickly our weights continue to increase compared to the number of workouts we've actually completed, it can be a huge motivational tool to stick with it.

PART IV:

EXERCISE NOTES

The "Breathing Paradox"

With everything else we've covered in regards to what makes this style of exercise so different, it should come as no surprise that breathing in regards to this style will be drastically different as well. For most people learning to lift there is a general rule of thumb for how lifting weights and breathing coincide: "Exhale as you lift, Inhale as you lower." This rule is extremely helpful when practicing traditional lifting; moving quickly in either direction. It serves little purpose however, when the course of your movements takes 4-12 seconds in either direction.

This same technique becomes completely inefficient while using the lifting outlined in H.2.L.G.N. You will find yourself very quickly out of breath, and over exerted. Therefore, for the purposes of moving slowly we will need to change the way we think about breathing in regards to lifting and lowering weights. When you move slowly throughout the course of a repetition and keep your muscles under continuous load it requires two things:

#1: More Blood

#2: More Oxygen

With the breathing you'll learn in H.2.L.G.N. you'll also accomplish two things:

#1: Getting your muscles the blood and oxygen they require

#2: Keeping your mind off the discomfort

The main thing we will be trying to accomplish when breathing through the course of our repetitions is to avoid something called "Valsalva". Essentially, that's just a fancy word for holding your breath. But any sort of breath holding (even if extremely brief) can raise blood

131

pressure, increase risk of stroke, and potentially lead to serious injury, or death. That might sound a little extreme, but most of the injuries I've seen that come from lifting weights, come from improper form and over exertion, which can be directly linked to breath holding (Valsalva).

When you stop breathing during bouts of extreme physical activity, even for a moment, you sap the oxygen from your blood which is already struggling to keep up with the increasing demands of the body. With no oxygen, muscles fatigue, focus lessens, and your ability to concentrate on things like form and safety go out the window. *Try this at home: Perform 10 air squats moving 10 seconds in each direction. First perform with only exhaling once on the way up and inhaling once on the way down. Second try the same 10 squats again, but breathing freely throughout the movement. Which is easier and more efficient?

So How Exactly Are We Supposed To Breath?

Ideally, while lifting in the H.2.L.G.N. program, we will get to a point where we are comfortable and proficient in practicing "proper and continuous breathing". The best way I can think to describe this style of breathing is something I would called "Controlled Hyperventilation". For those of you not familiar with the term Hyperventilation, think of any movie you've ever seen where someone breaths into a bag while having a "panic attack". Hyper (*meaning excessive or increased*) and ventilation (*literally just means breathing*), put them together and it's just a fancy way of saying excessive or increased breathing (I call it "over breathing"). There are a few tools you can also use to keep yourself safe and breathing consistent while exercising.

#1: <u>No Gum or Candy</u>: Don't workout with anything in your mouth. If you do, you drastically increase your chances of choking on something.

#2: <u>Loose/Relaxed Jaw & Face</u>: Try to keep your jaw and face as relaxed as possible. The idea of gritting your teeth and pushing through is a terrible one and tends to cause involuntary breath holding. Relaxed face = Relaxed Mind = Calm Body.

#3: <u>Breathing Only Through the Mouth</u>: This is far easier said than done. Breathing exclusively through the mouth serves a variety of purposes, but the main function is it's easier, and more efficient. Have water handy to prevent dry mouth.

#4: <u>No "Sound Effects"</u>: Grunting and groaning are sure fire indications that you are not breathing consistently. In order to make "sound effects" you must be exhaling, which means you are not inhaling, you want to be doing both.

#4: <u>A Little Dizziness is OK</u>: If you've never "over-breathed" before, the experience of doing so, especially in conjunction with the exertion involved in lifting heavy weights can cause you to get quite dizzy. This is harmless (though uncomfortable) and much better than the alternative of not breathing enough.

This concept once grasped is a huge stepping stone to making massive progress within the H.2.L.G.N. training program. That being said, like everything else in this book, it goes against a lot of the traditional information propagated in regards to training. Whether you know it or not, most of us have been conditioned to breath in a certain way, and that is our preferred method for however we choose to engage in physical activity. For traditional weight lifters it may involve lots of grunting, mixed with "exhale while you lift, inhale while you lower". For many clients I've trained who are yoga practitioners, it's extremely hard for them to get around their yoga conditioning of breathing almost exclusively through the nose. Just realize all those other styles may be well and good for the other things you choose to do with your time, but for the purposes of practicing this modality, this is not just the most effective way to breathe, it's the ONLY way to breath.

Before crossing the inevitable mental barriers that come with approaching failure in every exercise, the first major hurdle for most people is breathing. In my experience when you can begin to improve your breathing it serves as a tool to power you through those uncomfortable moments when your body is sending you every sign that you should stop. But once you see how you can literally "breath your way" to a few extra reps at what your mind was telling you was failure, it opens your eyes to how far you've come, and how much further you've got the ability to go. Don't Stop Breathing! Hold On To That Feeling!

It doesn't matter how experienced you are in this modality. When we get under extreme pressure and mental fatigue in the course of exercise, our brains begin to shut down. It doesn't matter how experienced or efficient my clients are, everyone's form begins to break and almost everyone forgets how to breath (myself included). This is when, especially early on, it's incredibly beneficial to have a trainer by your side to remind you to correct form discrepancies and to breath throughout the entire exercise.

For most of you beginning this program however, you will not have this option available. That's why it's so important to really work on your breathing early on in the training process, to prepare yourself for when things become increasingly harder down the road. A trick I like to use, and forgive me for getting this stuck in your head, is to imagine former Journey Frontman Steve Perry singing "Don't Stop Breathing", to the tune of "Don't Stop Believing", while I work through my routine. Occasionally this will trip me up and unconsciously force me to giggle, but for the most part it's a good reminder to keep my breathing consistent throughout the exercise.

Whatever tricks you need to use are fine, the main thing is to keep breathing no matter what. Even if you get dizzy, even if your muscles feel like they're going to explode, keep breathing, and you'll be amazed to see how much your body is capable of. For more tips on breathing, and what it actually looks like in the course of the movements, visit www.How2LookGoodNaked.com.

Form Discrepancies & Corrections

One of the main things to be aware of when it comes to safety in any type of new workout regimen is form discrepancies. The internet is full of dumb, unsupervised, or both, people who injure themselves in a never ending array of ways with different exercise equipment. The easiest target for these that I've seen seem to be Crossfit™ gyms. But really, it's anywhere people are doing large group training with complicated movements, time restraints, and limited sets of eyes. You mix those four elements together, and you are just asking for all sorts of trouble.

I firmly believe that you should not have to risk your health in any way, shape, or form, in order to work on improving it. This is why being aware of form and form discrepancies is so important. There is a difference between pushing your body past the point of discomfort, and getting to momentary muscle failure, and unfortunately this is hard to quantify for people. What you never want to see is people who are thoroughly exhausted and fatigued, pushing through in some vain showing of masculinity or dominance. Our bodies, just like with our diet, have given us certain innate cues to let us know we've reached our breaking point, you just have to be in tune with your body's messages.

To speak from personal experience (and in doing so shit on Crossfit™ a little more) there is a HUGE difference, between what I felt in Crossfit™ workouts for "failure" and what I feel using the H.2.L.G.N. method. The key difference is with H.2.L.G.N. I get to the point where I can no longer perform a rep with proper form or control. My muscles have failed in that moment (basically I'm stuck, and the only way I could get unstuck is to cheat). In Crossfit™, I would push well beyond this point of failure and get additional reps with any means necessary (I didn't try to cheat, I just cared more about additional reps and finishing than I did form).

As we know from earlier sections discussing the effectiveness of this modality, it's so effective because we never unload at *any point* during the course of the movement. In many Crossfit™ workouts (and a multitude of other group training environments) you are encouraged to take brief moments of respite and then get right back to it. What this ends up doing for those of us who want to take as little time off as possible, is compromise our form and our muscular integrity.

Yes, your muscles can recover extremely quickly when unloaded (to an extent), but at some point, the sand is falling out of the hour glass faster than you can shovel it in. When you get to that point, where you are trying to move heavy weight around and you reach true failure (not just MMF), your body does not care where you are in the course of a movement... it's gonna *shut shit down!*

One of the best parts about the H.2.L.G.N. method is that it's all machine-based training, which means your range of motion will be fixed to an extent, and it's much harder to injure yourself in the multitude of ways you can find by searching "Crossfit Fails". While being fixed in a particular plane of movement limits the potential for injury, it does not totally eliminate it. The biggest risk of injury in the H.2.L.G.N. method is from form discrepancies. The largest perpetrator of which is lower back stress and injury from arching, followed by shoulder strain and tension created by a variety of factors.

If you do these exercises correctly keeping form and breathing in line, this is as close to 100% safe as possible. You will still most likely experience muscle soreness at one point or another, but you should never feel like you've "hurt" yourself doing any of these movements. You can find examples of common discrepancies and videos to insure you are not displaying any of these on www.How2LookGoodNaked.com.

Environmental Concerns & Control

When I get new clients at any of my gyms they are consistently skeptical of two things:

#1: That they can get an effective, powerful workout in 20 minutes or less

#2: That they won't sweat while doing so

When dealing with clients in the initial consult and demo session, I'm not sure which one they believe less to start. However, when I take them back to the training rooms, though sometimes still skeptical about number one, they begin to see how number two just might be possible.

At my old gym, *My Strength Studio* in Minnetonka, MN they keep their training rooms at a frosty 62 degrees at all times. Along with that, they have heavy-duty personal fans at every individual exercise station, to cool clients down even more during the course of training. In the beginning this seems ridiculous, but the more you train in this modality, the more you begin to understand the importance of being cool while training.

Back when we discussed the "3 Reasons for Moving Slowly", reason number 3 was "Focus". Very few things break focus more than overheating, and when you do this type of training, you get very hot, very fast. The first time I tried the leg press at *My Strength Studio* I was *freezing* when I sat down, but I was also just learning the movement, and my intensity was not nearly as high. Now when I do the leg press I immediately turn the fans up to full blast. I know that I will be cold when I sit down, but I will warm up about halfway through the first rep, and be glad I have those fans on. This also allows busy clients to train in their work clothes. This means a large portion of the client base at *My Strength*

Studio comes in wearing a suit and tie, or a skirt and a blouse, and they train... in those clothes. It's a very alien concept to many of the new clients who come in expecting to have to wear "gym clothes", but they quickly grasp on to the convenience of not having to change their shirt or their dress socks.

As well as having climate control, *My Strength Studio* also has no mirrors, music, motivational posters, or anyone else to distract you while you are training. Everything is perfectly setup to make focus as easy and attainable as possible. You will most likely... not have any of that.

So exactly how the heck are you supposed to recreate those ideal conditions? For most people (especially those who can't afford a high-end gym like *My Strength Studio*) you won't be able to, but that doesn't mean you still can't create your own version.

Ideas For Creating You Own Ideal Exercise Environment:

#1: <u>Use music to drown out distractions</u>: while *My Strength Studio* keeps no outside music or noise (besides fans), when I workout with this method in other "regular" gyms I find music to be a necessity. For me it's Hip-hop, just loud enough so I don't hear whatever terrible Top-40 is most likely playing on the gym radio, but not so loud that I am consumed by it. Whatever your go-to workout music is, use that, but remember you're not there to "jam out", you're there to focus.

#2: <u>Having a timer available</u>: for most people the timer on your phone will be just fine. After a while you will find you don't really need a timer to keep your repetition speed in line, but it's still useful when you're getting to failure to record your total Time Under Load. I usually let the clock start and begin my repetitions when it gets to 20 seconds. This gives me a little time to mentally prepare for what I'm about to undertake, and also makes it really easy to subtract for my actual T.U.L. For static exercises do the same thing but add 10-20 second prep time before your 90-120s hold.

#3: <u>Stay cool at all costs</u>: the farther you get into this protocol the more you'll understand the value of staying cool. I used to workout in a full sweat suit because I assumed, *more sweat = better workout*. This is definitely not the case, and usually means the opposite. I still like to sweat, but now only in the sauna or a hot yoga class. Depending on how cool your gym is, consider wearing as light and loose of clothing as possible (shorts and a tank top if you've got it). As silly as it might seem, I would also recommend the addition of one of those old school water bottle/fans you find littered on the sidelines of youth soccer games. Especially if you tend to sweat or overheat as it is.

#4: <u>Map out your path</u>: in the on-boarding phase of this exercise program I talked a lot about knowing what you're going to do before you do it. This is really important to help eliminate distractions and make your workout as efficient as possible. When you get to the gym know what machines you're doing and in what order, and be ready to adapt on the fly. Having a backup plan will be supremely useful in keeping up efficiency and helping you in case some 70-year old dude decides to "camp" on the chest press for 10 sets. Also, be open to "working in" with someone if you have to. Remember, we've only got one set to do, if they open up the door to have us work in, they'll survive waiting once for up to 3-minutes.

#5: <u>Try to go solo, or with someone doing the same program</u>: I understand especially starting out, many of us want a workout buddy, and that's fine. If you do find it necessary to bring a partner in crime, try to make sure they're on the same page, and if possible, simply go alone once you get up to speed and feel comfortable with the protocol. Friends are great, gym friends are even better, but chit-chatting is one of the biggest distractions when you're trying to focus and be efficient and effective. You don't have to be a gym hermit, but if you wanna catch up, try to do it before or after your workout.

There's no perfect way to simulate the ideal environment, unless you're in a gym like the ones I've worked at, which are set up specifically for this type of exercise. For the rest of us however, using these simple tips will be extremely beneficial in helping you stay focused, get up to speed, and most importantly, start getting the results you want!

The "Cardio" Myth & Other Things We Hear That Just Aren't True

In the last part of this section I just wanted to take some time to dispel a few pervasive myths in the fitness industry. There are many people who will cry heresy at a lot of these claims, specifically because they've become part of the backbone of the financial structure of major fitness corporations. Nike™, Under Armour™, etc., these companies peddle certain fitness truths that are rooted in a long, rich tradition of misinformation. They are, however, completely without merit or real scientific evidence to support them.

If you'd rather go on living in ignorance (as we've already processed a lot of new information in these pages), you may want to just skip this section, and move onto the sample workouts, and dieting plan. If however, you are of the curious type and you want to see exactly what kinds of outlandish claims I plan on making, I'll give you a rundown of some of the Fitness Industry B.S. we are going to smash.

- The "Cardio" Myth: more specifically, that there even is such a thing as "cardio exercise", and that we've been led to believe the only way to improve aerobic capacity is jogging, cycling, ellipticals, etc.

- The "Calories In, Calories Out" Myth: examining diet and calorie counting, and why it's much more that just how much we eat vs. how much we burn.

- The "Plyometrics" Myth: the idea that plyometric training is safe and/or effective. That performing plyometrics somehow increases sports specific "explosiveness".

147

-    The "BMI" Myth: that simply by looking at someone's BMI (Body Mass Index) we can get a complete and accurate understanding of their general fitness level. This one is much more complicated than just height to weight ratio.

-    The "Scale Never Lies" Myth: this one is linked closely with the BMI myth and misinformation. The scale does in fact lie, and we'll explore a better and more accurate way of tracking progress.

Let's start with one of the most pervasive myths in the whole of the fitness industry, "Cardio". The following is another article written for clients and prospective clients at my former place of work. It's a little long winded (even by my standards), but I think it does a good job of explaining something that's very hard for fitness enthusiasts to come to terms with. "Cardio" as we have come to know it... is not real.

The "Cardio" Myth:
Un-inventing the Wheel:
Removing "Cardio" to Improve Cardiovascular Health

There are certain foundational beliefs that seem to be interwoven with modern health and fitness. Even people who don't know a dumbbell from a kettlebell seem to know these principles. It's as if they have been etched in the collective psyche of the masses.

"We hold these gym truths to be self-evident! That not all exercises are created equal."

Chief among these conceptions is the idea that in order to improve cardiovascular fitness, one must, without exception, work on and improve their "cardio". But what does this even mean? What is cardio, and why is

148

slaving away for hours on a treadmill, running 10k's and trekking for endless cycles to nowhere on an elliptical the only way to improve it?

If you take the blue pill, the story ends. You wake up in bed and keep thinking that the only way to improve endurance is to slave away endlessly on bikes, treadmills, and ellipticals. But, if you take the red pill, you stay in Wonderland, and I show you how deep the rabbit hole goes.

For most layman and even among many in the self-proclaimed gym elite, "cardio" is a foundational gym term. A building block upon which a true fitness enthusiast builds their home. This is why if you go to any gym in America right now you will likely see two diametrically opposed specimens participating in the same ritualistic pilgrimage to nowhere. Why is it that bodybuilders and distance runners practice the same way? Why is one trying to gain mass and the other is trying to stay lean, yet they both meet at this fork in the road in their training and take the path most traveled?

Let's look at the root of the word Cardio, Cardi, meaning "pertaining to the heart". So at the root of cardiovascular exercise is our heart. And how are jogging, cycling, and ellipticals meant to improve our hearts?

The heart, like many other misunderstood parts of the body, is a muscle. At its most basic, that's it, a muscle not unlike the biceps, quads, glutes, simply a muscle. Where the heart differs from other muscles however, is how it functions and what its main function is for our bodies. The heart is responsible for pumping blood, and life-giving oxygen to the rest of the body. But just like all other muscles in the body, it can only improve upon its functionality through proper, safe, and consistent exercise.

Where it all started to go wrong is with the introduction of a new word into the fitness nomenclature, something known as "Aerobics". The term Aerobics was first coined by Dr. Kenneth Cooper in the 1960's, and has since become wrongly synonymous with another word, Cardio. Dr. Cooper hypothesized and later advocated this idea of "Aerobic Conditioning" to the masses, and "Aerobics" as it would later be popularly known was born. Over the decades however, this misguided idea of Aerobics has become fused with the idea of "Cardio" and now the two are almost indistinguishable in how they are used in language.

While it would be ill-advised to argue that Aerobics under the guise of Cardio is inherently bad for one's health, it would be worse to consider Cardio as it is now defined "exercise". It simply is not. It is a recreational activity, and one who's pros and cons are beyond the scope of this piece. But, simply put, if improving your Cardiovascular System is one of your goals through exercise, you would be best served to stay away from anything under the guise of "Aerobics" or "Cardio Specific" exercise.

The simplest analogy for understanding the flawed logic of Cardio as we know it, may be as follows. Imagine that you have a goal to perform 100 10-lb dumbbell curls without stopping. Let's say when you first start you can only perform 20 of these curls without stopping. In order to increase your capacity for handling 10-lb curls which would make more sense? Should you continue to only curl 10-lb weights and hope for a slow steady improvement, adding a rep or two per training session? Or should you start with 20-lb dumbbells, and progress slowly and steadily to 20 reps with 40-lb dumbbells? The answer, without question is the second scenario. By increasing your overall strength with the 40-lb dumbbells with steady strength gains, when you are ready to try out 100 reps at 10-lbs, the weights will feel easy. This same logic can be applied to cardiovascular health, because the heart after all, is a muscle.

You see where Cardio, under the influence of Aerobics, goes awry is in the assumption that the heart can be isolated. This is not the case. If you want to improve the functionality of the heart, you have to improve the other muscles of the body. When our muscles become bigger and stronger, they require more blood and more oxygen. In order to increase capacity to the demands of the muscles' needs the heart must also become stronger and more efficient. This is why H.I.T. (High Intensity Training) is the gold standard when it comes to improving overall Cardiovascular Health. Just like our muscles respond, and grow to increased stimulus following the inverse relationship of Time/Intensity, so does our heart's capacity to pump blood and oxygen.

While this may seem counterintuitive at first, you can see the results and ramifications through sport, and almost all athletic competition. Most elite long distance runners will prep for a race by working "sprints" into their training. If you run 20 miles every day your body will wear down and be destroyed by the time competition arises. If however, you steadily increase your training to running 1,2, 4,8, etc. miles as fast as you possibly can, when the time comes to "pace" yourself, your body, and more specifically your heart are more prepared to handle this less intense exercise for longer periods.

The point is this. If increasing your "Aerobic Capacity" (i.e. Cardiovascular Endurance) is your goal, you will be better served by 20 minutes of High Intensity Training exercise, than continuing on the slow, steady, treadmill road to nowhere. If you enjoy Cardio, and it is part of your routine, then by all means, continue to do it. However, if you think the only way to improve your Cardiovascular Endurance is through endless hours of *spinning, ellipticals, and treadmills, rejoice, you now have a reason to get off the hamster wheel.*

Your Pal in Fitness,
Logan Herlihy
(Published December 2017)

    This first one stings for a lot of people. There are entire gyms and groups completely devoted to "Cardio Exercise". Again, this is not to say that you should never take a spin class or that running or walking isn't a great healthy hobby to have. However, aside from the science not actually adding up, there is another more pressing issue with people who are completely dogmatic about this Cardio idea. Specifically runners, more specifically, long distance runners.

    I'll tell you this now, and be as point blank as I can. Running for extended periods of time is potentially bad for you (due to associated risks; ankle sprains, bone spurs, etc.), but will probably not hurt you in the long run. Running consistently over the course of many years however, (i.e. career marathoners) is absolutely *catastrophic* on your body. It's arguably one of the worst things you can do to yourself (under the guise of exercise) if maintaining personal functionality late in life is important to you.

    There have been no scientific studies that I'm aware of that conclusively link running to an increased risk of osteoarthritis, in fact many show the opposite. As maintaining a healthy, active lifestyle which includes occasional recreational bouts of running can actually increase the longevity of knee and hip joints. The type of running I'm talking about is the fanatical kind. Those that run the equivalent of a marathon or more a week, for years, or decades.

Our bodies are extremely resilient machines, but they have limits. Long term exposure to consistent long distance running, is like exposing your body to a lifetime of Chinese Water Torture, and just trying to push off the moment when you finally break. To me, the risk is not even close to being worth the reward, but you can make up your own mind.

Again, I'm not opposed to running as a recreational activity, and even if it's on your bucket list to run a marathon, sure, go for it! But I would seriously caution anyone who wants to consider making a full-time hobby out of distance running. Crippling arthritis, blown tendons, micro fractures, multiple knee and hip replacements, that's what you have to look forward to when your running career comes to an end.

The "Calories In, Calories Out" Myth:
<u>Why You Shouldn't Drastically Restrict Calories,</u>
<u>Especially With Elongated Fasting Periods</u>

I'm not going to lie, this whole section is really going to mess with some people's heads. Even if you know *literally nothing* about dieting, most of us know some version of the idea that if you restrict calories, you lose weight. This idea is usually known as "Calories In, Calories Out". The thinking being that if you eat more calories than your body burns, you will gain weight, and if you eat less calories than you burn, you will lose weight. The problem is this is true... kinda, but it's much MUCH more complicated than that.

I am not nearly qualified enough to discuss the dynamics of metabolic processes, but there are a few things I do know from being in the health and fitness game for a while. One of the main things I've come to learn is that metabolism as we think we understand it is vastly more fluid and sensitive than most of us believe.

We live in the age of "Miracle Fat Burners" and "Metabolism Boosters", but the truth is as with most things involving diet, there is no consensus on what is 100% good or 100% bad for our body's metabolism. Things that were considered miraculous 5-10 years ago are now the targets of class action lawsuits (see: Ephedra), and things once considered metabolic killers somehow become miraculous (see: Bacon). This will continue to change and fluctuate, because the truth is, no one knows for sure what works and what doesn't. Sure we have ideas, but there's far too much fluctuation in human anatomy and biodiversity for a one-size-fits-all cure. So be wary of anyone who promotes such claims.

In this section I'll share with you some of the things I know (or think I know) about the metabolic process. Hopefully at the very least, we can erase some common misconceptions, most specifically, it's not nearly as simple as "Calories In, Calories Out".

Calorie Restriction and IM Fasting Don't Mix:

While the benefits of regular intermittent fasting have been widely reported and studied, what many people wrongly assume about IMF is that fasting means not eating. Which let's be real here, that's literally *exactly* what it means, but fasting also means *feasting* in the eating phases. What trips many people up when they first begin a protocol of IMF or Time Restricted Eating, is they end up unintentionally (sometimes intentionally) restricting calories as well. While some other diets may be proponents of limiting calorie counts, that is not the case at all with H.2.L.G.N. If you're eating the right types of nutrients, in the right time frames, the calories should take care of themselves, and you shouldn't have to strictly keep track.

Occasionally when following a regular IMF protocol, you will restrict your calories, just from pure circumstance. Certain days I'm too busy to eat as much as I would like, sometimes my fast goes on extra long and I just forget, but for the most part I eat more than most people my size would consume, and I don't even feel a little guilty.

What happens when we start to drastically restrict calories within a IMF protocol is that in the beginning you will see rapid weight loss. Your body is already running more efficiently due to the IMF, and you're burning more calories than your consuming, it's a double whammy. But what happens to people who take this approach in my experience is that after initial success, they *very quickly* hit a wall, where their body will no longer allow them to lose weight, gain muscle etc.

This often leads to people wrongly thinking they've plateaued and that they must restrict calories even more! Usually what happens after this is great amounts of frustration followed by people either staying where they are, or even *gaining weight*. They assume that IMF simply does not work, or they've got a thyroid issue, or whatever it might be. However, the reality as strange as this may sound to some is usually that they were not *eating enough to lose weight!*

When we restrict our calories past a certain point, especially while already incorporating IMF in combination with a modified Keto/Paleo diet, our natural survival instincts begin to take over. Our bodies (hardwired from generations of famine at some point in history) switch to conservation mode and our resting metabolism slows down to a crawl. The body begins to store any available calories or metabolic resources in the fat department to be used at a later time, and if carried on long enough with also begin to eat away at muscle tissue (muscle has much higher metabolic requirements and as such becomes unnecessary in times of famine). So in an attempt to lose weight and "be healthy" many people get stuck when they find not only are they no longer losing weight, they are also losing muscle and strength.

This is one of the dirty secrets about fad diets that continues to keep new people coming in, but also results in the cycle of losing then regaining weight for SO MANY people. If you restrict calories, you *will* lose weight, if you restrict them for too long or too often, you will put that weight right back on. It's no wonder most diets under the vein of "cleanses" or "whole body change" only last 30-days or less. If you keep starving yourself after that time frame, your results won't be nearly as effective.

The most obvious example of this would be contestants from the television show, "The Biggest Loser". The show follows contestants who lose massive amounts of weight over the course of filming (many times 100 pounds or more). Though most people will not experience the drastic metabolic changes associated with the caloric restriction and exercise routines the contestants go through, it shows us something very important about metabolism. The vast majority of the contestants end up gaining the weight back, and sometimes even more weight.

But why, if calories are controlled and their weight has gone down? The reason it seems is that our bodies don't like be threatened with the idea of starvation. After the drastic diet and exercise overhauls the contestants experience, their resting metabolic rates plummet. Meaning someone who now weighs 180 pounds only burns enough calories to maintain a weight of 130 pounds. So over time (even with restricting calories) they inevitably put all the weight back on. For those doing H.2.L.G.N. this simply means that we are taking the long game approach to diet and exercise. Being smarter about *when* and *what* you're eating, may not help you lose 100 pounds in six months, but it will prevent you from short circuiting your metabolism in the long run.

So What Should I Do Instead?

Total body/lifestyle change takes time. It's not something you can accomplish in a 30-day challenge, or even a 3-month boot camp. It takes dedication, persistence, and most importantly... time. If you are or used to be in shape, your results may be drastic and rapid as your body adapts faster to old habits. If however, you have not changed your diet or participated in regular exercise in a long time or ever, this isn't going to happen over night. The thing to remember is that if you stick with it, and follow this protocol, you shouldn't have to feel cheated out of foods you enjoy eating, and your physiological changes will come with time. Instead of trying to lose "a pound a day" like some diets claim, why not stay consistent and shoot for a pound a week or every two weeks. At the end of 12-months you'd be down 26-52 lbs, and with that kind of slow consistent effort, you'll most likely stay down for good.

If your diet seems too good to be true, it probably is. Even with the diet outlined in this book I saw *incredible* results quickly (almost 15 lbs lost in two weeks), but since then its become a lifestyle, and one that I've come to enjoy immensely. I haven't lost much weight since then (most likely my body has found an ideal weight at 6 feet and 165 lbs and achieved homeostasis), but I also haven't gained any, and I've had the opportunity to enjoy what I'm eating on a daily basis, and spoil myself to the extreme whenever I see fit.

The Plyometrics Myth:
Why Jumping on Boxes Will
Never Equate to Better Sports performance

I'll be honest with you, this next one hurt a little bit. I was not ready to give up on the idea of plyometrics and dynamic sports-specific training, but the evidence just does not support the claims. For those of you that are not familiar with plyometric training, the idea is essentially this; to apply maximum power and exertion through a movement for a minimal amount of time, in order to increase strength and "explosiveness". Think box jumps, dynamic bounding exercises, explosive push-ups, etc.

This type of training modality became exceedingly popular in the late 90's and early 2000's (when I was active in team sports), and still is a foundational practice in many CrossFit and other H.I.I.T. style training facilities. While there are still many trainers who swear by incorporating plyometric training into their routines, the evidence has never quite come to support the theory.

The reason (at least as far as I can tell) that plyometrics became such a popular choice of trainers is because logically, it makes sense. Basically, the idea is that if you "Train fast/train explosive" you will play faster and with more explosion (makes logical sense). The main draw of plyometrics was that it would increase an athlete's "explosiveness" (think tackling for football players or dunking for basketball players). As it turns out however, explosiveness, like many other dynamic traits certain athletes might possess, is not actually coachable. Basically, you can do box jumps all day, but if you don't have the natural physical gifts to throw down a dunk from the foul line (a la Jordan 1988), no amount of training, plyometric or otherwise will get you there.

This is where plyometrics, like many other types of fad training have missed the mark over the years. People don't like to hear this next part (so if you're feeling extra sensitive, cover your eyes), but the truth is... nothing, no amount of training, or heart, or guts... NOTHING trumps genetics. Plyometrics and its popularity is partially to blame because of those advocating for it... athletes, coaches, and trainers.

Think about it this way. If you take the top 1%, of the top 1% of the world's athletes, and put them on a specific training modality, they will almost always excel and get some sort of benefit from it (real or perceived). What plyometrics actually train you to do by jumping on boxes is to get really, really good... at jumping on boxes. However, when we see someone like Lebron James incorporating box jumps into his workout, and telling us how much box jumps have helped his game, we assume that if we only started jumping on boxes... maybe... just maybe.

Plyometrics is not the only offender, this has happened for probably as long as sport has been around and we've wanted to emulate our favorite athletes. Normally fitness fads come and go, and I wouldn't even spend any time picking out a particular "myth" within them to discuss. The reason we're discussing plyometrics more than others however, is because aside from being ineffective, plyometric exercise is also inherently dangerous and reckless behavior. This becomes especially compounded when you start incorporating it into routines with novice clients, and inexperienced/unprofessional trainers. Don't believe me?

159

Google "Box Jump Fails" and go travel down that wormhole for a little while.

This all goes back to our modality and training style in H.2.L.G.N. Which some might argue is too simple, or not challenging enough. I can assure you, you do not need to do crazy shit to have a powerful and effective workout. And compared to plyometrics, which has an exceptionally high level of injury risk, the methods I have outlined in this program have as close to no risk as humanly possible (without being able to actually say it for the sake of liability).

There's an anecdote I read while putting together this book from a *SuperSlow* training advocate in the 1990's. At a convention in a hotel where they were discussing *SuperSlow* training, before going on-stage to speak, he was informed that someone had recently jumped from the top floor of the hotel to their death. Upon hearing the news this particular advocate simply said to his crowd, "Someone needs to tell these guys that they are taking this Plyometrics thing a little too far."

The BMI Myth:
Why We Shouldn't Put Too Much Weight(lol)
On the Body Mass Index in Regard to Overall Health

This myth is pretty straightforward and to the point, and something that I just wanted to help clear up for some of my readers who may not be familiar. BMI or Body Mass Index, is a general equation used in the health and fitness industry to determine an individual's general baseline physical health. The confusion with this one comes in because BMI does not account at all for physical activity, diet or lifestyle. It's simply an overarching baseline which uses a height-to-weight ratio to determine which zone a particular client falls within. Essentially, this is how it is setup:

BMI
BMI $\leq$ 18.9 = Underweight
BMI 19-24.9 = Healthy Weight
BMI 25-29.9 = Overweight
BMI 30-39.9 = Obese
BMI $\geq$ 40 = Extremely Obese

So, for instance, if you are a 6'0" man between 140-180 pounds, you would fall in the "Healthy Weight Category". Then a different 6'0" man at or above 230 pounds is considered "Obese", and any weight in between there would fall under the "Overweight" category. This is a great general overview of what range you should be in, but just realize that this is not a perfect system. For instance, you could take those same two 6'0" individuals, one at 180 pounds the other at 230 pounds, and just basing what we know off BMI you may assume the first man is in better shape. This is where we have to have a basic understanding of BMI to know that this is not always the case.

If for example, your first man is highly sedentary, working a desk job, with little to no physical activity, he may only have a BMI of 24, but his body fat percentage and skeletal muscle mass could be completely disproportionate. The second man however, with a BMI over 30 may in fact be a bodybuilder or a football player with an extremely low body fat percentage and extremely high skeletal muscle mass.

It's because of this that BMI is not the most effective tool for those who are new to dieting or exercise. It gives you an extremely broad understanding of where you potentially fall along the bell curve of fitness. But in order to create a plan of action, we're going to need much more detailed information than what BMI can offer. Which happens to be a perfect segue into our last myth...

The Scale Never Lies Myth:
Weight is Important, But Not That Important
When It Comes to Tracking Our Progress in Diet/Exercise

Just like with BMI, our weight is a major topic of contention when it comes to exactly how it is a reflection of our progress in any new diet or exercise program. Everyone's metabolism and body types are extremely different and their relationship with a scale can vary drastically. Some of us shed weight whenever we start a new program, and while this can be exciting, it may not always be a *good* thing. Others of us can seem to just look at certain foods and put on extra pounds regardless of our efforts in the gym or in the kitchen.

What we're trying to accomplish with this book is a total body change and overhaul, but at a slow and steady pace. Some of you might experience incredible weight loss within days of starting Intermittent Fasting, others may not notice any significant weight shift right away. The thing we're trying to explore with dispelling this particular myth, is that neither of those are inherently bad. What we should be looking for, after an initial period of adjustment is to start *feeling better*, this is how we know we are making progress. Weight loss will come with time, but if we are attempting to achieve a healthy body and lifestyle that we can most importantly easily maintain, that takes time. We'll be erasing and eradicating years (or sometimes a lifetime's worth) of bad habits, and that's not something that just happens overnight.

The scale is a valuable tool, but not always to be trusted. Like I stated in the beginning of this book, before I started this program it was not uncommon for me to fluctuate upwards of ten pounds *per day!* Today my daily weight rarely fluctuates more than 2-3 pounds depending on how long I've been fasting, and how badly I was cheating the night before. What's more valuable than simply looking at our weight, is something that goes a little deeper into our actual physiological changes, our plan for this is twofold.

Step 1: Take Pictures. In the beginning I would recommend once per month for up to 3 months, and then only quarterly (every 3 months) thereafter. The reason for this is over exposure. We see ourselves, every day, and because of this we are oversaturated with ourselves. When you look in the mirror every morning it's next to impossible to track the small changes in our appearance that happen on a micro basis every day. To the outsider however, these changes slowly start to add up. Remember for a second, a time when you have run into someone that you hadn't seen in a while. Someone that had either lost or gained a drastic amount of weight. To you, the change seems obvious.

But to the person, it happened so slowly (whether good or bad) they most likely were not aware of it until others started to point it out. The same thing happens with us, and is the reason many people get frustrated and give up on a program. They spend too much time looking at a scale, and not enough time comparing how much their physical appearance has actually changed.

Step 2: Use a Body Composition Tool. There are a variety of tools for tracking body composition, which is drastically more important and useful than weight or BMI alone (DEXA, BodPod, and BIA's). Essentially these machines track your actual physiological makeup in regards to body fat, lean muscle mass, body water, and some even offer a segmental lean analysis (comparison of how your muscle composition stacks up against the average). While DEXA and BodPods are rarer, many gyms offer complimentary services of high-quality BIA's, such as Inbody.

You can also sometimes find these services available at doctor's offices or therapy offices. What makes these machines so valuable, is they show you an actual breakdown of how your body is changing from the inside out. Just like with pictures, when used quarterly, you can track progress on a much deeper level, and really see the differences you may not otherwise notice. The key is to pick one tool for measurement and stick with it. Your results from a BodPod to a BIA may be different, but if you use the same BIA you should be able to track progress over time.

If, for instance, you were our same 6'0" male from earlier on day one with a BMI of 25 and a weight of 180 lbs, you may be discouraged six months later to find that your BMI is still 25 and your weight is still 180 lbs. If you are just using a scale to track progress, you might feel like giving up at this point. If you had been tracking your progress with a BIA and pictures however, you might notice that in that time your body fat decreased from 20% to 15%. This means in six months that you experienced not just a loss of 9 pounds of body fat, but you also gained 9 pounds of muscle, for an *18 pound* swing!

By using pictures, you would also be able to compare yourself from day one, and see the drastic changes that a significant drop in body fat and gain in muscle mass has on you. Even though your weight is the same you would have smaller hips, tighter muscles, and a firmer more chiseled physique. Without the use of these tools, these drastic changes you've made - and should be celebrating - might have gone unnoticed, simply due to your own overexposure to yourself.

There's plenty more myths out there, but they are beyond the length and scope of this particular endeavor. What I hope you see from the few covered here however, is that almost nothing in the gym is written in stone. What we think we understand about fitness and nutrition is really just our best guesses at the time. The problem is some of these ideas that we should have learned were wrong, stick around for far too long. Anyone who says they have figured exercise and nutrition out is lying to you. That's why I'm not claiming this is the only way to get in shape, this is just the easiest and most efficient way I've found so far. If something better comes along, I'll jump on that bandwagon, but to date, this has given me by far the most bang for my buck.

All we truly know is that exercise is good for us, and proper diet can have huge positive or negative effects on us depending on what we choose to eat, when, and how. Beyond that, no one knows for sure, and most of the information was collected just as much by dumb luck as by actual research. I would encourage everyone who reads this to give my methodology a shot; take what works and leave the rest. I would also encourage you to be wary of anyone who proclaims to know better. We are constantly bombarded with promises of grandeur and the many "magic bullets" of new and exciting fitness and nutrition. That "magic bullet" does not exist. There are however, many well educated people who will disagree with some of the things I've outlined in this book, and I honestly could care less about those people. H.2.L.G.N. is about two things 1. Feeling Great and 2. Looking Good, and in my experience if you take care of number one then number two will always follow.

In the final section of this book, we're going to be outlining a plan of action; getting started, tracking progress, and sticking to it. So at this point you've finished the meat of this book, the rest is how to put this new information into action. It's been a pleasure getting this far with you all, and I hope at this point you're ready to commit a minimum amount of time and effort, in order to make a maximum change. I wish you all the best of luck on your journey, and I hope to hear your stories of struggle and ultimately success along the way!

PART V:
INTO ACTION

Making a Plan

We've made it this far and it's finally time to start taking some actual steps to get this thing moving. In the beginning, our first objective was to simply start becoming aware of *what* and *when* we're eating. Now we're going to start putting that information to use. What this last part of the book is about, is essentially breaking down a general 3-month outline for you to slowly start incorporating all these ideas into your daily routine. Like I've said from the beginning, the more ideas in here you can incorporate, the more effective this program will be. Without rushing, three months should be more than enough time for everyone to start making small changes, see some results, and continue to keep building.

That being said, you can start this thing off with a bang right now if you want. Simply making the "Zone 1: Least Restrictive" ideas part of your daily life will be hugely effective for most people. As far as I'm concerned, the more you wanna do, the better! But for those of you that have problems with retention, that have a history of getting "burnt out", go as slow as you need, we're making massive changes here, and there's no rush. What you need to do though is hold yourself accountable, if you plan to ease into this thing, that's fine, but don't continue to push it off. If you plan on adding something by the end of the first month, add it. The only thing worse than trying too much too fast, may be stagnating in diet "limbo" for six months and wondering why you're not seeing any results. Here's a general idea of what this process over the course of the next three months should look like:

Month 0-1:

- Getting blood work, and finding foods to avoid

- Recording our starting point using Body Composition Tools, photographs, and also BMI, and weight (the last two as reference points)

- Starting to incorporate general Intermittent Fasting principles, as well as a daily practice of the gut "window" (minimum 12-hours between last and next meal & eating for less than 12-hours/day)

- Trying to fast for 12-16 hour a few days a week (and planning the day before, what and when you'll eat)

Month 1-2:

- Starting to focus more on the *what* that we're eating (limiting sweets, starting to eat higher fat foods)

- Incorporating the "Zone 1: Least Restrictive" ideas on a regular basis (strict adherence to the gut window, limiting carbs to less than 150g every day, etc.)

- Starting to cook for ourselves on a regular basis, and creating a catalog of delicious recipe ideas (I highly recommend www.ketodietapp.com), and becoming extremely aware of what we eat when we "eat out"

- Starting to research places we could begin our exercise program. There's no need to be exercising regularly yet (if that's not already part of our normal routine). Try to find a gym that will be accommodating to our workouts when the time comes (if you already belong to a gym, begin to identify the proper equipment we'll be using)

Month 2-3:

- Rarely if ever straying outside of "Zone 1:Least Restrictive" ideas, and starting to incorporate "Zone 2: Moderately Restrictive" into weekly routine (gut window <10 hours, limiting carbs, limiting eat out, etc.)

- Going deeper into identifying when we are in Ketosis

- Starting the process of *Phase 1: Groundwork* in the exercise protocol (identifying equipment, building charts, starting to go through the motions of the workouts)

- Building a solid foundation of creating our own meals, and getting more comfortable and working with our own personal Intermittent Fasting window

Month 4 - beyond:

- Recording our first (quarterly) progress report before we get too deep into the exercise protocol. Body Composition Tools, photographs, BMI and weight. Continue this quarterly going forward.

- Up to *Phase II: Getting Acclimated* in the exercise protocol at this point, and continuing through the rest of that program

- Extremely comfortable and in a rhythm with our daily diet at this point, creating personal accountability and continuing to add and incorporate more beneficial ideas from a range of sources.

The next section in this book will be the final before we wrap this whole thing up. We're going to delve a little farther into what this outline will look like when applied to our real lives. I'm going to give you some suggestions for things you should try to do, before, during, and after this experience (though hopefully a lot of these principles are things you will carry over). There are a few things we will clear up as far as dietary restrictions and how those might affect you with this program.

The main thing here is listening to your body. As I stated before, many of us are not aware of the subtle signals and warnings our bodies are naturally designed with. By being more aware of what we're putting into our systems we'll start to become more aware of these subtle, but important signals. There is no *one diet* that's better than all the rest. This form of Ketogenics and Intermittent Fasting has been extremely beneficial for me, but that doesn't mean it's the only way of achieving success. That being said, there are many other diets under the guise of "optimal health" with proclamations of superiority that don't seem to be aware of this underlying principle that not a single one of us is exactly the same.

Vegans love to proclaim the health and wellness benefits of a plant-based diet, and while the immediate impact of switching from highly processed foods to an entirely plant based diet is profound, the long-term success of such diets are just not supported scientifically for most people. Vegans have done a wonderful job of creating awareness in the food industry, but the "holier than thou" approach they take turns many people off to what can be a great way to jumpstart your metabolism and immune system. The reality is that most people need animal products of some kind in the long run, even in small doses.

Meat, and the essential proteins and fats it provides are vital to immune system regulation and proper maintenance of hormonal and cellular function. That doesn't mean you should just eat meat with reckless abandon. We should definitely be conscious of the foods we are eating and where they are sourced, but with some of the steps outlined in the next section we will discuss some ways to find out what our *ideal diet* should look like. This is based on a variety of factors, including but not limited to, food allergies, sensitivity to foods, current gut biome makeup, and genetic predisposition to certain dietary requirements.

Sticking to It

This is a diet and exercise plan made for the person who wants to look as good as possible, with the least amount of effort. That being said, there are plenty of little "add-ons" we can incorporate in this process to help make it as smooth and painless as possible. The first of which we've discussed many times is *going slowly* and not trying to change too much, too fast. The following section also includes some other helpful tips, that are by no means required, but can definitely assist in this process of getting up to speed, and optimally tracking results.

#1: *Getting a blood test/testing for food allergies:* This goes a little bit more into understanding exactly what our bodies *want* us to do. Getting a blood test will allow you to see where you are deficient as far as minerals are concerned, and will also give you a chance to talk to your Doctor about the new adventure you're about to undertake. Getting tested for food allergies is vitally important in my opinion for most people whenever you attempt to drastically transform your eating habits. Many of us have allergies and sensitivities to certain food groups (gluten, dairy, etc.), which if eaten in the course of trying to change our diet, can totally ambush and destroy our efforts. Simply by being aware of certain foods we may be sensitive to, is enough for many people to start seeing changes in how you look and feel. (I would highly recommend seeing a homeopathic nutritionist for these tests as opposed to a straight-laced doctor. As we've already discussed many in the medical field are stuck in archaic forms of methodology, better in my humble opinion to find someone who is willing to support you and think outside the box).

#2: _Gut Biome:_ This one is invariably related to the first recommendation. The preponderance of evidence coming out of late in the dietary community is that many of the problems in this country linked to obesity and disease are related to a blatant disregard to our guts. If you go so far as to seek out a medical professional for blood work and food allergies, I would strongly advise also talking to that person about what steps you can take to jumpstart your gut biome. This is one of those topics where I am vastly under qualified, but a good starting place would googling some of Dr. Rhonda Patrick's' findings about the gut biome, and getting yourself on a potent probiotic. While the web is an excellent tool for reviews and finding the best probiotic for you, the following are a few helpful starter tips. Look for a probiotic with upwards of 10 + strains of bacteria (multiple patents), and upwards of 10+ billion live cultures.

#3: _Getting a Body Composition Test (DEXA, BodPod, BIA) and taking some "before" photos:_ We already covered this one pretty extensively, so I won't go too far into it, but for the sake of tracking _real progress_ these two things are invaluable. The BIA (or whatever tool you use) will show us how we are changing from the inside out from a physiological perspective. The before photos serve as a great tool to use as a measuring stick for our outward progress along the journey.

#4: _Making a realistic fasting schedule:_ Before we even begin the process of actually incorporating fasting into our daily routine it helps to start thinking what this schedule might look like down the line. For women, I would recommend you fast for 12-16 hours (usually only 12-14) when you are actually in the swing of things. For men, I recommend 16-22 hour fasts (usually only 16-20) when you get up to speed. Try to get an idea of what your day may look like before you begin to attempt this.

Assuming a man and woman both work a typical 9-5 workday the two fasting schedules when starting out might look something like this:

Woman 12-hour: Waking up at 7 am (after last meal at 7pm night before), can immediately start with a cup of coffee with butter and MCT oil (12-hour gut window has been met, and she is free to eat throughout the day) and probably having her first high-fat meal around 10am and finishing by 7pm that night. In this case the 12-hour gut window has been met 7pm-7am, and the minimum 12-hour fasting window has also been met.

Woman 16-hour: Waking up at 7am (after last meal at 7pm the night before), can immediately start with a cup of coffee with butter and MCT oil (12-hour gut window has been met, but still needs 4 additional hours of "fasting"). From 11am on she can eat throughout the day until her last meal at 7pm that night. In this case the 12-hour gut window has been met 7pm-7am, and by waiting till 11am for food (supplementing with coffee) the 16-hour fasting window has also been met.

Man 16-hour: Waking up at 7am (after last meal at 7pm the night before), can immediately start with a cup of coffee with butter and MCT oil (12-hour gut window has been met, but still needs 4 additional hours of "fasting").From 11am on he can eat throughout the day until his last meal at 7pm that night. In this case the 12-hour gut window has been met 7pm-7am, and by waiting till 11am for food (supplementing with coffee) the 16-hour fasting window has also been met.

Man 22-hour: Waking up at 7am (after last meal at 7pm the night before), can immediately start with a cup of coffee with butter and MCT oil (12-hour gut window has been met, but still needs 10 additional hours of "fasting". Most people cannot go this long, especially at first.

And you shouldn't be fasting this long on a regular basis. Coffee will keep you alert, but I would recommend with longer fasts stopping coffee at or around noon. Too much caffeine past this time can disrupt your sleep schedule. If you feel you must have something to satiate you, try a hearty caffeine free tea with butter and MCT oil for later in the day). From 5pm-7pm he can indulge in all the high-fat goodness he can stuff his face with. In this case the 12-hour gut window has been met 7pm-7am, and by waiting till 5pm for food (supplementing with coffee) the 22-hour fasting window has also been met.

This is where the gut window starts to come into play, remember initially we just want to limit food intake (and anything that's not water) to 12-hours throughout the day (eventually 9-10), or at the very least give our bodies 12-hours between the last thing that's not water we put into our bodies, and the next time we put something that's not water in. These examples regardless of the fasting window are all using the 12-hours on/12-hours off principle for our gut. As you get more comfortable you will begin to either push your first cup of coffee until later in the day, or have you last meal finish earlier in the day.

By doing this you are shrinking the gut window to less than 12-hours and giving your body the most available time to break down, process, and be ready for work again the next day. In real life this may fluctuate from day to day, which is why it's important to have a general awareness of how these time frames work. If I'm up early for work on a day (say 5am), I already had my last meal by 5pm the previous night. This means when I wake up I've given my gut the minimum of 12-hours. If I have my coffee at 6am, and I want to try to stay under the 12-hour gut window cap that day, I know I will have to have my last meal that day by 3-5pm (9-11 hours of gut time).

Assuming I finish eating at 4pm that day, the next day when I wake up at 8am, I will have already fasted for 16-hours by that time, and I can now feel free to eat under the 12-hour gut window until 8pm that night. It's a constant give and take, but the most significant results you will see are influenced by limiting your gut window, even more so than fasting. So make 9-11 hours of anything "not water" your priority.

By no means are these things all required. Again, take what you want and leave the rest, but with any new diet or exercise program I feel these are all things that should be included. Preparing yourself before you even take the first step is a great way to ensure retention when things get hard. If you've already battled with the ups and downs of scheduling before you've even picked up a weight or looked at a scale, you're *way ahead* of the game. The ideas outlined in this section are just to give you that extra leg up, and even by just doing those things alone, and becoming aware of what types of foods you're eating you're at a huge advantage over everyone else.

These ideas are there to help inspire you, and make you want to stick with it! If you've been allergic to gluten your whole life and have never known, that could be the thing holding you back. That fact alone mixed with a few ideas in this book, might be all you need to start reaching the goals you've always had for yourself. Give this thing a shot, stick with it, and I think you'll be surprised at the results.

Summary & Personal Results

Before we wrap this thing up, I just want to take a moment to remind you of a few things that are the backbones of this program. At the root of this program is only one central and primary goal, I want you to feel good, no better than good, *great!* Even if this whole thing seems a little intimidating at first, remember at the end of the day, it's all about you, and making you feel the best you've ever felt. You don't have to do all of the things I've outlined in these pages to feel better, these are just all the things I've found easiest and most effective for myself.

More than anything what I hope to create with this book is a conversation. I want people (like you) to start questioning the status quo. To not just take things at face value. My hope is that this will be the jumping off point for you, and help inspire you to not just take my word for it, but start doing some research of your own. Like I said in the beginning, if you do *some* of the things in this book, you'll get some results, if you do all the things, you get *great* results. But don't take that to mean that this is all there is. For you this might just be the beginning. Use these methods, start feeling better and looking better, and then go find something custom made and tailored exactly to your specific needs. Only *you* know what the ultimate you looks like.

The truth is, after many years in and out of the gym, I'm perfectly content with my current system. I turned 30 this year and I want to continue my fitness journey, but currently maintaining a healthy and low-maintenance physique is ideal for my lifestyle. This doesn't mean in two years I won't all of a sudden get the urge to pack on 30 pounds of muscle again (I don't see that happening, but you never know). If that becomes the case then my dietary and exercise habits will probably shift... again. This information I've shared with you however, is something that has become the bedrock of my fitness plan. I don't have to waste hours on Cardio anymore (and I never will again); I don't have to slave away endlessly 2-hours a day at the gym. These realizations have been life changing. What I want more than anything is to be healthy, and to me that means only two things:

#1: I want to feel great

#2: I want to look good

As long as those two foundational requirements are met, I could really care less about how I achieve those goals. I hope that you have found what's in these pages to be helpful, and at the very least found a few new interesting things you might want to try. I mentioned in the beginning there is no monthly membership plan at the end of this trip, but I do want to make myself available to anyone that may have questions, concerns, or simply wants to talk a little more in-depth about health and nutrition.

Make no mistake, I do not have all the answers. I know less than many, but more than most. What knowledge and insight I do have I want to make available to anyone kind enough to purchase this book. If you have found anything in here you would like to discuss in further detail please reach out to me. My email is logan@how2lookgoodnaked.com. Please don't hesitate to contact me and share your experience, good or bad.

Lastly, I want to wish you all the best of luck in your fitness journey. It's a long, arduous road, but the juice is most definitely worth the squeeze. We only get one life, and we only get one body. It's in our best interest to try and take care of it.

I've made a lot of claims and done a lot of talking about the amazing results I've seen while developing this program. In this last little portion here I just wanted to take a moment to share some of those actual results with you, the reader. You can find all of this information and more on my website:

www.How2LookGoodNaked.com

The following are some of my personal BIA's as well as before and after pictures in my training with this program.

I want to hear from all of you, I want to share your stories and experience your journey with you. Please reach out with before and after pictures of your own on www.How2LookGoodNaked.com to spread your experience, your own struggles and victories, recipes, workout ideas, etc. My goal is to help build the most courteous and caring fitness community on the web, with incredible results from incredible people. I look forward to hearing from all of you!

Your Pal in Fitness,
Logan Emmett Herlihy

"The best time to plant a tree was 20 years ago, the second best time is now."
-   Chinese Proverb

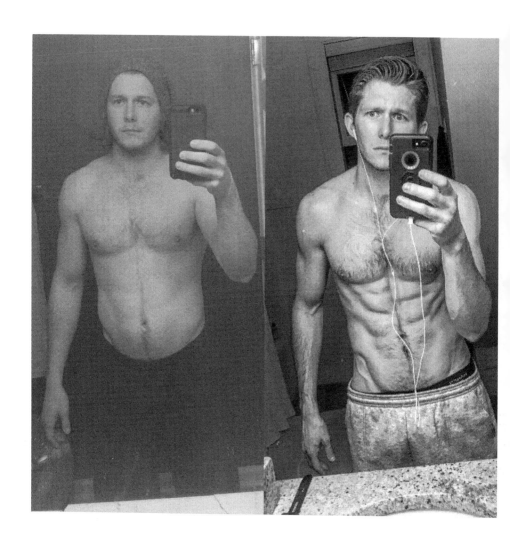

Logan's Results (From 12/17-8/18):

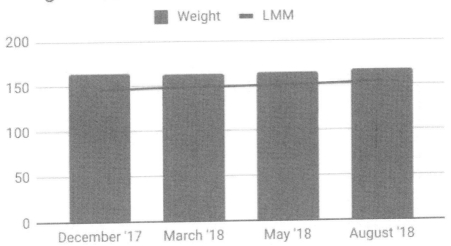

187

Body Fat %

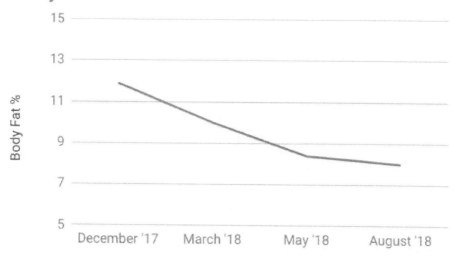

Skeletal Muscle Mass

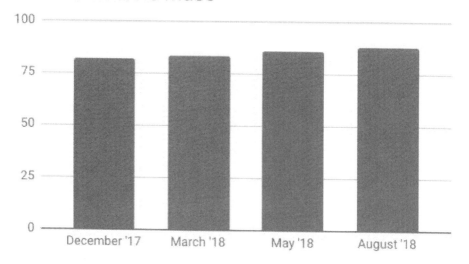

APPENDIX

Naked Coffee Recipe

- 8-12 oz hot coffee (personally I make my own cold press and reheat it)

- 1-2 tbsp grass fed butter (Kerrygold is my favorite)

- 1 tbsp High Quality MCT Oil (*Bulletproof©, Onnit©, etc.*)

- 1 large dash of Organic Turmeric Powder

- Mix all ingredients in a blender (*Magic Bullet©, Ninja©, etc.*) and blend until frothy, around 30s.

- Dump into coffee cup and enjoy :)

Workouts: Exercises & Modifications

H.T.L.G.N "BIG 5" WORKOUT ROUTINE

1. LEG PRESS

2. SEATED SUPINATED GRIP PULL-DOWN

3. SEATED CHEST PRESS

4. SEATED PARALLEL GRIP COMPOUND ROW

5. SEATED OVERHEAD PRESS

CHEST PRESS MODIFICATIONS:
1. STATIC CHEST PRESS (90-120S)
2. DECLINE/INCLINE PRESS
3. SUPERSLOW PUSH-UPS
4. SEATED CHEST FLYS
5. RESISTANCE BAND CHEST PRESS

Compound Row Modifications:

1. Static Compound Row (90-120s)
2. Bent-over DB/BB Row
3. Seated Resistance Band Row
4. Weighted Compound Holds (90-120s)

Leg Press Modifications:

1. Static Leg Press (90-120s)
2. Leg Extension/Leg Curl (Dynamic)
3. Static Leg Extension/Leg Curl (90-120s)
4. SuperSlow Air Squats
(Body Weight/Weighted)
5. Wall Sits (Body Weight/Weighted)

Overhead Press Modifications:
1. Static Overhead Press (90-120s)
2. DB Overhead Press Holds (90-120s)
3. Seated Delt Raises
4. Simple Row
5. Seated Overhead Press w/ Resistance Bands

Pull-down Modifications:
1. Static Pull-down (90-120s)
2. Weighted static hold (90-120s)
3. Limited range Pull-down
4. Resistance Band Pull-down
5. Assisted Supinated Pull-up

Workout Tracker Outline:

Workout #1	Seat/Settings	Notes	(Date of Workout)
(Machine Type) Exercise [sequence #]	Seat 2, Seatback3	Injuries, ROM, etc.	Weight/Reps (Time)
(Hammer Strength) Seated Calf Raise [1]	N/A	Watch stretch at bottom ROM	100/10 (120)
(Nautilus) Trunk Extension [2]	Seat 2, Pad 3	Limited ROM at bottom, progress slowly	90/8 (115)
(Hammer Strength Leg Press [3]	Seat 5, Back 3	Left Knee issue, stop reps at 10	250/9 (150)
(Life Fitness) Pulldown [4]	Seat4, Neutral Grip bar	Rotating Neutral and Supinated grip	120/14 (140)
(Cybex) Horizontal Handle Chest Press [5]	Seat 3	Watch shoulder impingement at bottom	140/10 (90)
(Hammer Strength) Seated Row [6]	Seat 2	N/A	120/8 (140)
(Cybex) Overhead Press [7]	Seat 3, Pad 2	Watch shoulder impingement at bottom	80/10 (120)
Exercise Notes:			

H.2.L.G.N. CHARTS: QUICK REFERENCE

Zones of Eating:

Zone 1: Mildly Restrictive (7 days a week):

- *Limiting my gut intake (circadian rhythm) to 12 hours or less per day*
- *Fasting for at least 12 hours every day*
- *Including some type of healthy fat in every meal*
- *Limiting sweets and processed foods whenever possible*
- *Never consuming more than 150 grams of net carbs in a day (holidays and special occasions excluded)*
- *Avoiding fast food whenever possible*
- *Minimizing Alcohol Consumption*

Zone 2: Moderately Restrictive (4-7 Days a week after being in Zone 1 for a month)

- *Limiting my gut intake to 10-11 hours a day*
- *Fasting for up to 12+ hours (women) or 16+ hours (men) every day*
- *Limiting my carbohydrate intake at every meal (less than 75 net carbs/day)*
- *Avoiding eating out more than once a day, saving money and more in control of nutrients*
- *Drinking alcoholic beverages (no more than two, no more than twice a week)*

Zone 3: Majorly Restrictive (3-5 days a week after being in Zone 2 for a month)

- *Limiting my gut intake to no more than 9-10 hours a day*

- *Fasting for up to 18+ hours every day*
- *Monitoring carb intake (keeping to less than 50 net carbs/day)*
- *No sweets, no sugar, no "fun" stuff*
- *Keeping a 70/25/5 (fat/protein/carb) ratio throughout the day (keto)*
- *At 2,000 calories per day, this means 150/125/25 grams (fat/protein/carbs)*
- *If that math looks wrong, it's because fats have a higher caloric content (9 calories/gram, compared to 4 calories/gram for protein and carbs)*
- *Preparing my own meals, and portioning appropriately for the week*
- *Completely abstaining from alcoholic beverages*

Assumed vs. Real Objective:

Assumed Objective:
- Quantitative Approach
- Increase Metrics (sets, reps, weights, etc.)
- Goal to make all metrics go UP

Real Objective:
- Qualitative Approach
- Achieve Inroad/MMF every time
- Goal: Stimulus -> Body -> Adaptation

H.2.L.G.N. Training Curve:

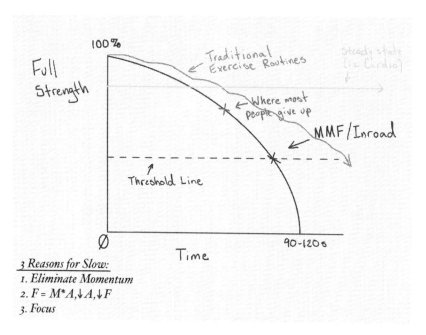

3 Reasons for Slow:
1. *Eliminate Momentum*
2. $F = M*A, \downarrow A, \downarrow F$
3. *Focus*

Time/Intensity Principle:

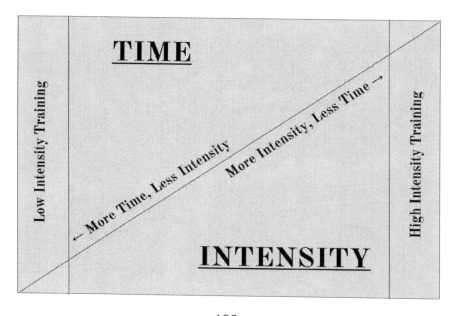

Fasting Schedule:

Women's 12-hour Fasting:

- 12-hour gut window has been met, free to eat Keto throughout the day
- Last meal finished by 7pm at the latest that night
- 12-hour gut window and 12-hour fasting window has been met

Women's 16-hour Fasting:

- 12-Hour gut window has been met, still need 4 additional hours of "modified fasting"
- 1st Keto meal at 11am or later, last meal by 7pm or earlier that night
- 12-hour gut window and 16-hour fasting window has been met

Men's 16-hour Fasting:

- 12-Hour gut window has been met, still need four additional hours of "modified fasting"
- 1st Keto meal at 11am or later, last meal by 7pm or earlier that night
- 12-hour gut window and 16-hour fasting window has been met

Men's 22-hour Fasting:

- 12-hour gut window has been met, still needs 10 additional hours of "modified fasting"
- Eating as much high-fat and Keto friendly food from 5-7pm as possible
- 12-hour gut window and 22-hour fasting window has been met

Made in the USA
Lexington, KY
08 November 2019